EATING FAT WILL MAKE YOU FAT

This edition published in 2018 by André Deutsch
An imprint of the Carlton Publishing Group
20 Mortimer Street
London W1T 3JW

First published in 2017 under the title *Myth-busting Your Body*

10 9 8 7 6 5 4 3 2 1

A CIP catalogue record for this book is available from the British Library.

ISBN 978 0 233 00572 0

Printed in Dubai

EATING FAT WILL MAKE YOU FAT

AND OTHER HUMAN BODY MYTHS BUSTED

Dr Sarah Schenker

ANDRE
DEUTSCH

CONTENTS

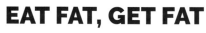

INTRODUCTION

MYTHS ABOUT DIET AND nutrition have always been around, but I feel there has been a surge in recent years. Media attention to diet has also exploded, so it can often feel as if we are living under a huge blanket of conflicting and contrasting advice about what we should and shouldn't eat. Diet fads come and go, as do celebrity "experts", but our enthusiasm for the latest diet trend never wanes. In addition, there is much more coverage of nutritional science in the media, with, for example, studies on the effect of oily fish on conditions like Alzheimer's often making the front pages of national newspapers. By contrast, studies from other areas of scientific research hardly ever make it into the newspapers.

All this isn't surprising – we all make choices about what we eat, and we know that what we choose impacts on not only our health but also our day-to-day experiences, be it our mood or physical performance. Yet nutrition is a complex science and often it is oversimplifying this science that paves the way for dietary myths. Many of the most popular dietary creeds are myths, not backed by any scientific evidence, and even, in some cases, contradict the existing body of evidence. These myths can become obstacles to people making the best dietary choices, despite the fact that they are seeking to improve their diet or health status.

Dietary myths surround everything from caffeine to so-called "superfoods", but most attention focuses on diet and weight loss. This is to be expected as the obesity epidemic and diet-related conditions such as type 2 diabetes envelop the Western world. The increase in obesity cannot be explained by a sudden shift in our genetics, so it has to be down to the huge changes in diet and lifestyle habits that have occurred over the last hundred years. And yet as we have become on average fatter, the social pressures in relation to body image have increased. There is no doubt that the fear of gaining weight in today's society has contributed to the proliferation of diet and nutrition myths and a rise in the popularity of fad diets, "miracle" products and the promise of magical results.

But should we be worried? Aren't most myths just misleading rather than harmful? Unfortunately, a common theme in dietary myths is elimination of food groups. Just think of dairy-free, gluten-free or carb-cutting diets, to name a few. Many of these fashionable diets can lead to inadequate intakes of essential nutrients and make health worse rather than better. In almost all cases, dieticians would advocate the rather boring and unsexy approach of consuming all foods in moderation – a health choice unlikely to make headlines!

I think it is important to dispel dietary myths and misinformation on food in particular for the younger generation, who face the prospect of increased risk of ill health with rising rates of obesity and a lack of adequate nutrition. A healthy, well-balanced diet is key to the maintenance of general good health and wellbeing. In order for people to understand this we need to develop engaging educational campaigns in the field of nutrition. I hope this book goes some way to explaining away the most commonly held myths, and showing you why it's important to do so.

Dr Sarah Schenker

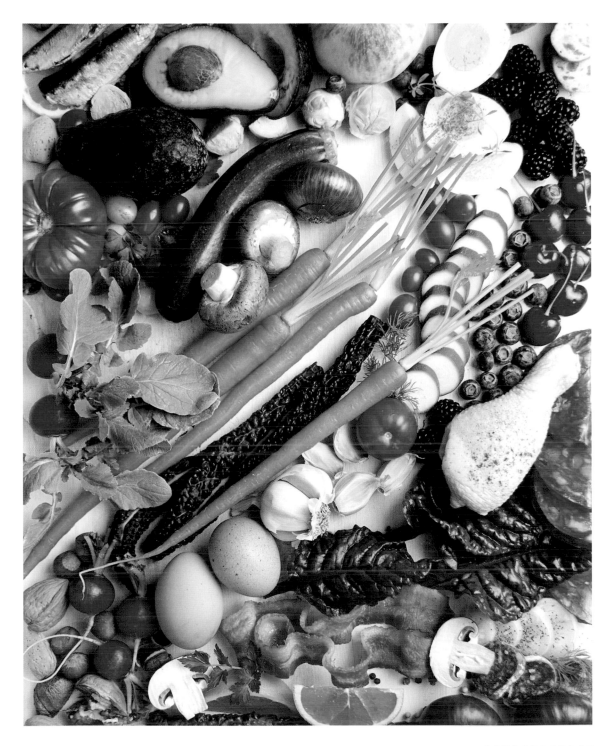

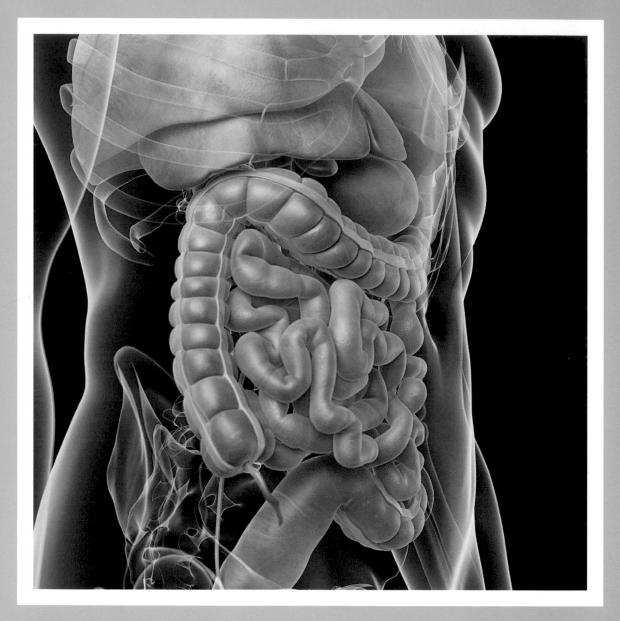

1

GUT FEELINGS

Myths relating to digestion, gluten, dairy and probiotics

THE DIGESTIVE SYSTEM: AN OVERVIEW

Digestion is the process of breaking down food to release nutrients, which the body uses for energy, growth and the repair of cells. Food and drink contain large molecules (such as protein) that must be turned into smaller molecules (such as amino acids) before they are absorbed into the bloodstream and taken to cells throughout the body, where they are needed for various biological processes.

THE DIGESTIVE SYSTEM CONSISTS of a series of organs, each of which plays its part in the conversion of food into nutrients that are essential for good health. The nutrients are absorbed into the body and anything left over unused is eliminated as waste. Our bodies depend on the daily provision of adequate amounts of nutrients, and on being able to eliminate waste products that can otherwise be toxic, so health can be compromised when the digestive system does not work properly.

Each section of the digestive system is controlled and regulated by nerves and hormones that trigger what are known as homeostatic mechanisms, which feed back to the gut and make subtle changes in absorption rates. For example, during pregnancy, hormones signal the gut to absorb larger amounts of minerals such as iron and calcium, which are needed for the growing foetus. While these hormones stimulate the production of digestive juices and regulate appetite, nerves help control the

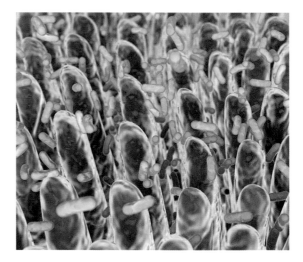

ABOVE: The gut flora of the human digestive system is a complex community of microorganisms which includes "friendly" bacteria that can support good health.

action of the digestive system and release chemicals that speed up or delay the movement of food and the production of digestive juices. Gut bacteria (also called gut flora or microbiome) are another crucial part of the digestive process. These healthy bacteria are necessary to properly digest food and absorb nutrients.

The digestive system is made up of the gastrointestinal (GI) tract, also known as the digestive tract, and the liver, pancreas and gallbladder. The GI tract is a series of tubes joined to form one long, convoluted tube; it comprises the mouth, oesophagus, stomach, small intestine, large intestine (including colon and rectum) and anus. The entire system from mouth to anus is up to about 9 metres (30 feet) long.

The digestive system

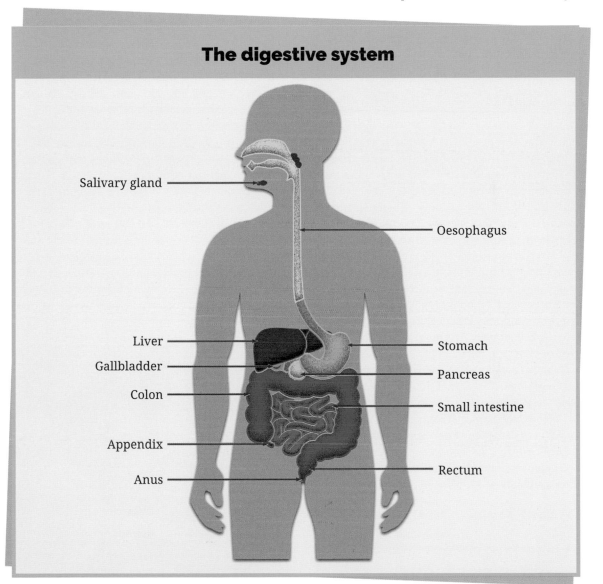

Salivary gland

Oesophagus

Liver

Stomach

Gallbladder

Pancreas

Colon

Small intestine

Appendix

Anus

Rectum

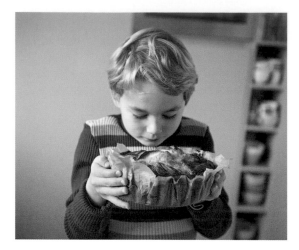

The digestive process can start almost as soon as you smell or even think about food. The release of saliva in the mouth is the first stage. Saliva plays two roles: it moistens food to make it easier to form a ball, known as a bolus, and it contains an enzyme known as salivary amylase, which starts the breakdown of starch in food. Chewing and grinding food are also important for forming this soft bolus.

Swallowing pushes the bolus into the oesophagus, where it passes through the oropharynx and hypopharynx in the throat. At this point you cannot help but continue, as the action becomes involuntary. The oesophagus, like other parts of the gut, is made up of rings of muscle that contract and relax in a rhythmic sequence, squeezing the bolus further down towards the stomach. This process is known as peristalsis.

The lower oesophageal sphincter, a ring-like muscle at the junction of the oesophagus and stomach, controls the passage of food and liquid. As food approaches the closed sphincter, the muscle relaxes and lets it pass through to the stomach.

....

ABOVE: The smell of food increases the secretion of saliva, which lubricates the food we eat.

RIGHT: A cross section of the human stomach and small intestine.

The stomach then releases gastric juice, which is a mix of hydrochloric acid and the enzyme pepsin. Pepsin starts to break down proteins into peptides and amino acid, while the hydrochloric acid kills potentially harmful bacteria. Food will stay in the stomach for two to three hours and eventually form a thick paste known as chyme.

Once chyme has been formed, the muscle at the bottom of the stomach, called the pyloric sphincter, opens and the chyme enters the duodenum, the first section of the small intestine, where it mixes with more digestive enzymes released from the pancreas and also bile acids from the gallbladder. The pancreatic enzymes are responsible for the further breakdown of carbohydrates as well as fats and proteins. The bile acids are needed for the breakdown of large fat molecules into smaller molecules that can be absorbed.

The chyme then passes into the ileum (the last section in the small intestine), where most of the nutrients are absorbed. Specialized cells help absorbed materials cross the intestinal lining into the bloodstream, which carries sugars, amino acids, small fat molecules and some vitamins and minerals to the liver. The lymphatic system, which is connected to the gut (an everyday term for the

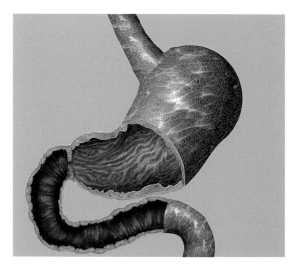

gastrointestinal tract), absorbs fatty acids and other vitamins.

The liver creates glycogen from sugars and carbohydrates to give the body energy, and converts dietary proteins into new proteins needed by the blood system. The liver also breaks down unwanted chemicals, such as alcohol, which is detoxified and passed from the body as waste.

Whatever material is left goes into the large intestine, this part of which is known as the colon. The colon is approximately 5 feet (1.5 metres)

long and its primary function is the storage and fermentation of indigestible matter. The colon has four parts: the ascending colon, the transverse colon, the descending colon and the sigmoid colon. In the colon, some of the water from the chyme is absorbed back into the body and faeces are formed from remaining water, dietary fibre and other waste products, including older cells from the GI tract lining. Muscles push the faeces into the rectum and they are stored here until they are eliminated from the body through defecation.

TRUST ME, I'M A DIETICIAN
Looking after your digestive system

A rich meal or an extra-spicy curry (accompanied by one too many glasses of alcohol) is unlikely to give you anything worse than a short-lived stomach upset. But overindulging too often can cause problems of heartburn, constipation or diarrhoea.

Eating more fibre is key to preventing chronic constipation. Most people fall short of the recommended dietary intake of 25g to 30g (c.1oz) per day. For a healthy bowel, you need fibre from a variety of sources, such as wholemeal bread, brown rice, fruit and veg, beans and oats.

Fluids are also important for digestion, so it is important to drink regularly – especially water, as it encourages the passage of waste through your digestive system and helps soften stools.

It is crucial to increase your intake of both water and fibre, because they work together: the fibre acts like a sponge, absorbing the water, without which stools will be hard and difficult to pass.

Indigestion and heartburn are usually related to eating too much. The stomach stretches after a big meal and produces more acid, which can either irritate the stomach lining or rise up into the oesophagus. This irritation can be painful and cause a burning sensation. Spicy and fatty foods and fizzy, alcoholic and caffeinated drinks can all aggravate heartburn.

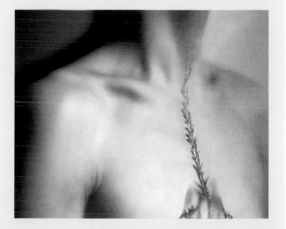

DO FOOD COMBINATIONS AFFECT THE DIGESTIVE SYSTEM?

Many years ago it was suggested to dieters that their weight problems weren't to do with how much they ate, but rather lay in the combination of foods they ate at each meal.

FOOD-COMBINING DIETS SUCH as the Hay diet recommended that protein and carbohydrate foods should not be eaten together, because each hindered the digestion of the other and this poor digestion of food somehow caused weight gain or prevented weight loss. Foods were divided into three categories: protein foods, such as meat, fish and dairy; neutral foods, such as fruit and veg; and starchy foods, such as cereals and grains.

The rationale behind the advice to not combine protein with starch is a belief that when protein-rich foods are consumed, the body produces too much acid to digest starch, for which an alkaline condition is needed. Conversely, the digestion of starch results in there being too little acid present to kick-start the digestion of protein. To date there has been no scientific evidence to support this theory.

More recently, food-combining has taken on a new dimension, focusing on acidic and alkaline foods. The alkaline diet is one of the breakout diets of the last few years, promising to improve

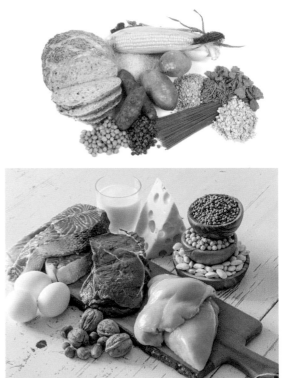

energy levels and memory as well as help prevent headaches, bloating, heart disease, muscle pain and insomnia. Supporters of the diet claim that almost all foods we eat break down into either an acidic or alkaline base. Fresh fruit, vegetables, roots, nuts and legumes are all good. Dates, figs, grapefruit, lemon, lime, fennel, broccoli, artichoke, asparagus, beetroot, kale, spinach, watercress and cauliflower are considered the most alkaline. But pasta, wheat, all dairy products, meat, fish and shellfish, coffee, tea, sugar, fizzy drinks and alcohol are all seen as acidic and therefore out. Considering the health benefits and low energy density (i.e. calories per gram) of the "good" alkaline foods, it is unsurprising that such a diet would aid weight loss.

There are also bold claims that cutting out acidic foods and sticking to a mainly alkaline-based diet can help prevent a range of medical problems including osteoporosis, arthritis, diabetes and cancer, as well as slowing the ageing process. One popular message among the trendy bloggers is that dairy is actually bad for your bones because it is acidic.

Certainly it is clear that the pH (scale of acidity) and acid load in the human diet has changed considerably from the hunter-gather civilization to the present. With the agricultural revolution and industrialization, our diets have seen a decrease in potassium compared to sodium and an increase in chloride compared to bicarbonate.

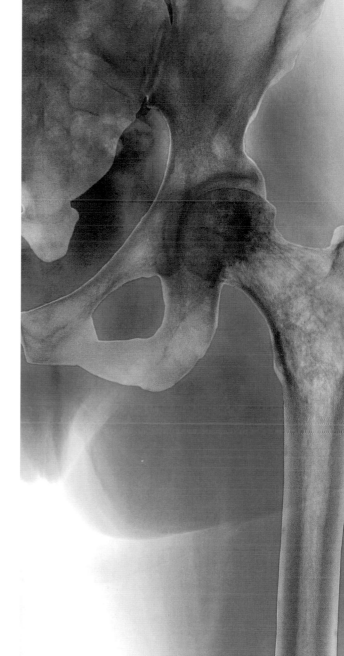

OPPOSITE ABOVE: *Examples of foods high in carbohydrate include pasta, bread and potatoes.*

OPPOSITE BELOW: *Examples of foods high in protein include meat, eggs and dairy products.*

RIGHT: *It is claimed that acidic foods can increase the risk of poor bone health, evident in this hip joint showing osteoporosis.*

The bicarbonate buffer system

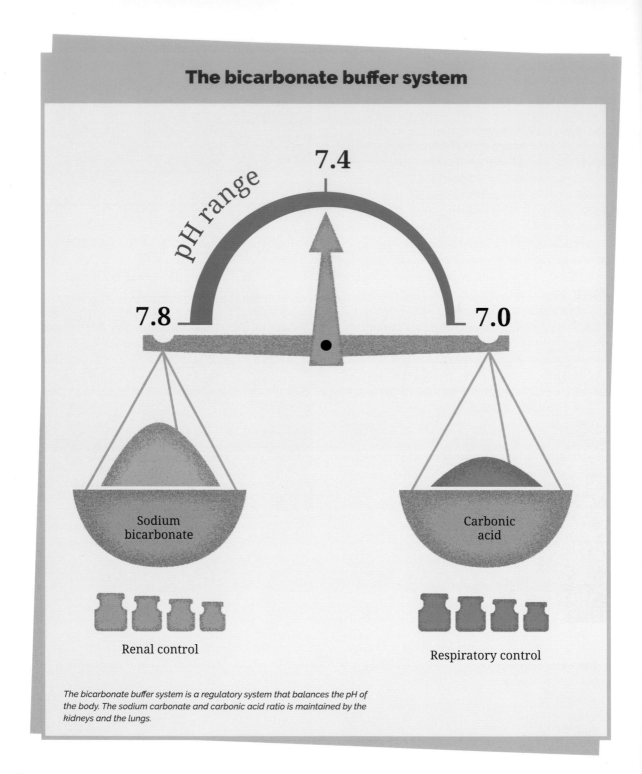

The bicarbonate buffer system is a regulatory system that balances the pH of the body. The sodium carbonate and carbonic acid ratio is maintained by the kidneys and the lungs.

The ratio of potassium to sodium has reversed: previously it was 10 to 1, whereas the modern diet has a ratio of 1 to 3. It is generally accepted that today we have a diet poor in magnesium, potassium and fibre, and too high in saturated fat, simple sugars, sodium and chloride. However, the claims that such changes can result in metabolic acidosis are unfounded. Instead, the human body has an amazing ability to maintain a steady pH in the blood through the compensatory mechanisms that occur in the kidneys and through respiration. This process is known as the bicarbonate buffer system (see diagram on page 16). With ageing, there is a gradual loss of this regulatory function and popular low-carbohydrate, high-protein diets can increase the acid load, but even in such circumstances there is very little change in blood pH. Instead, changes occur in the urine where the lower pH may be a risk factor for kidney stones.

Our pH levels vary considerably from one area of the body to another, with the highest acidity in the stomach (pH of 1.35 to 3.5) in order to aid in digestion and protect against opportunistic bacteria. The skin is also quite acidic (pH 4–6.5) in order to provide an acid mantle as a protective barrier against microbial overgrowth.

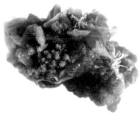

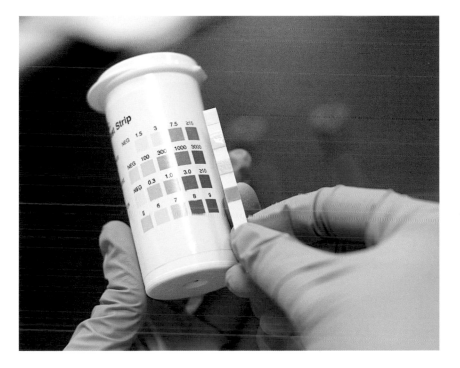

ABOVE: Kidney stones are caused by a build up of crystallized waste products from the blood that collect in the kidneys.

LEFT: A urine pH level test measures the acidity or alkalinity of your urine and can be used to determine risk of kidney stones.

The bottom line: Urine has a variable pH, from acid to alkaline, reflecting what the body has been doing during digestion to balance itself. On this basis, foods can be categorized by their potential acid loads and so alkaline diets will result in a more alkaline urine pH and may result in reduced calcium in the urine, but this does not impact on bone health and there is no substantial evidence that an alkaline diet improves bone health or protects from osteoporosis.

IS GLUTEN BAD FOR EVERYONE?

Bloggers, vloggers and self-styled "nutritionists" (without qualifications) preach about the toxic effects of gluten, declaring it the root of all health problems, such as weight gain and mood swings. It's a wonder how something we have been consuming for thousands of years has become the scourge of the twenty-first-century diet.

THESE CONCERNS, WHICH GO on to be propagated by the press, Internet and social media, have led to some wild claims, unsupported by conventional medical evidence. The impact has been dramatic – not only on wheat producers and the food industry but also on public health, due to the effect on our intake of nutrients conventionally consumed in wheat products, such as dietary fibre, B vitamins and minerals.

WHAT IS GLUTEN?

Gluten is the main storage protein used by some classes of flowering plants to nourish seeds during development and germination. The protein is found in grass-related grains, including wheat, barley and rye. It consists of two classes of protein, a glutelin and a prolamin (known in wheat as glutenin and gliadin, respectively). The prolamin components of gluten help wheat to form dough by creating a viscous elastic network. That's why high-quality gluten flours produce the best bakes.

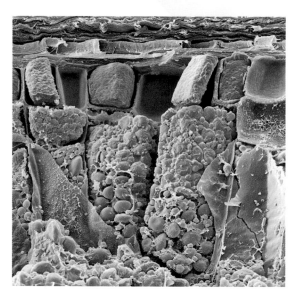

ABOVE: A cross section of a grain of wheat, showing the store of starch grains (yellow) below a layer of cells containing protein (green).

HISTORY OF GLUTEN

Cereal crops became a component of the human diet about 10,000 years ago during what is known as the Neolithic Revolution. This saw a transition from the hunting and gathering of food to settled agriculture. Cereal harvesting and consumption have steadily increased since then. The improvement of wheat cultivation became a focus of Western countries and today global wheat production amounts to over 700 million tonnes per year.

The need to ensure the efficient agricultural production of wheat has led to artificial breeding of

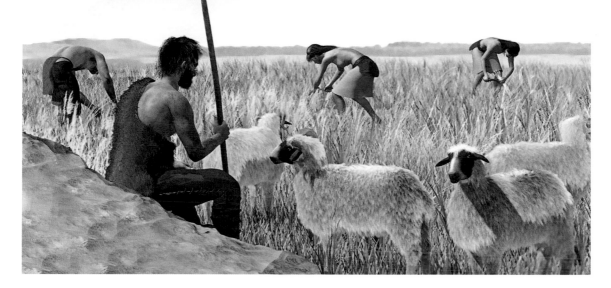

wheat variants better adapted to extreme climate conditions, also selected for their bread-making qualities and resistance to diseases. Currently, about 95% of the wheat grown worldwide is bread wheat (*Triticum aestivum*), a hybrid of an ancient species and a wild grass species. It is favoured by farmers for its superior qualities and yields. It is also popular in the baking industry as its increased gluten content is better for bread and cakes, which rely on its elastic and stabilizing abilities.

There's an argument that gluten exposure has increased too quickly to give our immune systems the time needed to develop and adapt, and that this in turn has caused the rise in coeliac disease and other gluten-related disorders.

WHAT IS A GLUTEN-RELATED DISORDER?

Gluten-related disorders have been classified into three broad categories:

- allergic reactions, such as a wheat allergy;
- auto-immune disorders, which include coeliac disease, dermatitis herpetiformis (a skin condition) and gluten ataxia (a neurological condition);
- immune-mediated disorders, in the form of non-coeliac gluten sensitivity.

ABOVE: We have been harvesting grain crops since Neolithic times.

BELOW: A normal section of the small intestine (top) and a section affected by coeliac disease (bottom). Flattened villi reduce the capacity of nutrient absorption.

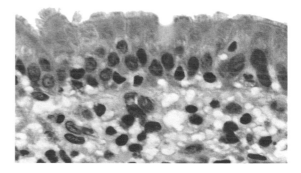

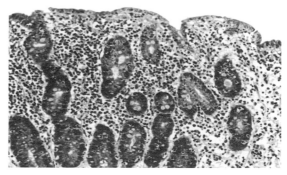

Coeliac disease is a chronic inflammation of the gut lining caused by ingesting gluten. It is now estimated that 1% of the worldwide population has coeliac disease. It is also widely accepted that a considerable proportion of patients still remain undiagnosed, with estimates that, for every patient diagnosed with coeliac, approximately eight cases are yet to be detected. And, while it was once believed to be a disease of childhood, adult cases are now far more frequent.

Symptoms of coeliac disease such as failure to thrive in a child, chronic diarrhoea and weight loss are relatively rare. Patients are more likely to suffer irritable bowel syndrome (IBS), iron deficiency anaemia, osteoporosis and neuropathy.

IBS is common, affecting about 10% to 15% of the world population. International guidelines recommend that all patients presenting with IBS should be tested for coeliac disease. To date, the only treatment for coeliac disease is a lifelong gluten-free diet.

GLUTEN INTOLERANCE

Gluten intolerance, or non-coeliac gluten sensitivity, causes gastrointestinal and other symptoms triggered by the ingestion of gluten-containing food, even when coeliac disease has been ruled out through blood tests and biopsy. The symptoms include abdominal pain, diarrhoea, constipation and bloating, as well as chronic fatigue, behavioural changes, bone or joint pain and muscle cramps. Symptoms typically occur shortly after the ingestion of gluten, stabilize on a gluten-free diet and relapse after consuming gluten.

The condition is often self-reported but can be confirmed by medical diagnosis using the presence of what are known as anti-gliadin antibodies (substances produced by the immune system to attack gliadin protein) as a test positive. The growing awareness of gluten intolerance has led to increased investigation of the pathology and mechanisms of the condition. However, there is of course controversy.

One of the biggest confounding factors for diagnosing gluten intolerance is the efficacy of

Antigens and antibodies

Pathogens such as viruses and harmful bacteria contain certain chemicals that are foreign to the body, called antigens. Once an antigen enters the body, the immune system destroys it. Although the proteins in wheat are not pathogens, sometimes the body thinks they are harmful and triggers the immune system to destroy them in the same way.

White blood cells are important components of the immune system, as they produce antibodies to destroy antigens. White blood cells called lymphocytes carry the antibodies that have a chemical "fit" to a certain antigen. When a white blood cell with the appropriate antibody meets the antigen, it reproduces quickly and makes copies of the antibody so that the pathogen can be neutralized again. However, in the case of food in the gut this repeated process can cause damage, resulting in the symptoms of gluten intolerance.

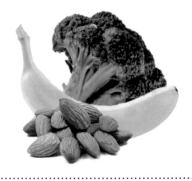

ABOVE: The restrictive nature of the FODMAP diet means that even the healthiest of foods need to be avoided.

avoiding FODMAP foods. FODMAP stands for fermentable oligosaccharides, disaccharides, monosaccharides and polyols – basically foods that are poorly absorbed in the gut – and a low-FODMAP diet is used to successfully control IBS symptoms. This has led to the suggestion that components of wheat other than gluten may be responsible for triggering IBS symptoms. For example, FODMAPs such as fructans, largely found in wheat and related grains, can trigger gastrointestinal symptoms.

Studies have shown that individuals with gluten intolerance on a self-imposed gluten-free diet show further improvement when placed on a low-FODMAP diet and that the subsequent reintroduction of gluten has no effect.

GLUTEN-FREE DIETS

The number of people consuming gluten-free diets now greatly exceeds even the highest estimates of those suffering from gluten-related disorders. For many, the avoidance of gluten is viewed as a "healthier lifestyle" change rather than as treatment for an actual disorder.

Consequently, the scientific community has had to acknowledge this trend and consider the wider impact of gluten-free diets on nutrition and health.

TRUST ME, I'M A DIETICIAN
Bread alternatives

Not all breads are the same and if you experience discomfort or bloating or other bowel problems when you eat bread, rather than choosing a gluten-free variety, try a traditionally made sourdough. Although wheat has been part of our diet for centuries, the digestive problems associated with bread have increased rapidly since the 1960s. This coincides neatly with the invention of the Chorleywood bread process – a technology breakthrough behind over 80% of the bread available in shops today. The traditional method for making bread requires flour, water, natural yeasts, salt and plenty of time for kneading and proving. Time of course is money in the food industry, and the Chorleywood process uses all sorts of additives and enzymes to reduce the production time. Traditional bakers may ferment their dough for days to produce a "ripe" dough fizzing with lactic acid bacteria, or lactobacilli. As a result of skipping the fermentation process, modern bread does not contain these beneficial lactic acid bacteria, which have a number of benefits: they can improve the bio-availability of minerals in the bread, meaning they are better absorbed by the body, and lower the glycaemic response (which is better for weight and diabetes control). Most importantly, scientists have now demonstrated that sourdough lactobacilli are capable of neutralizing the gliadin fractions in the wheat flour that are toxic to coeliacs and people with similar sensitivities.

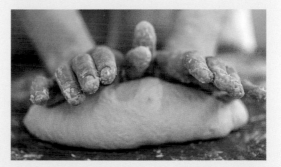

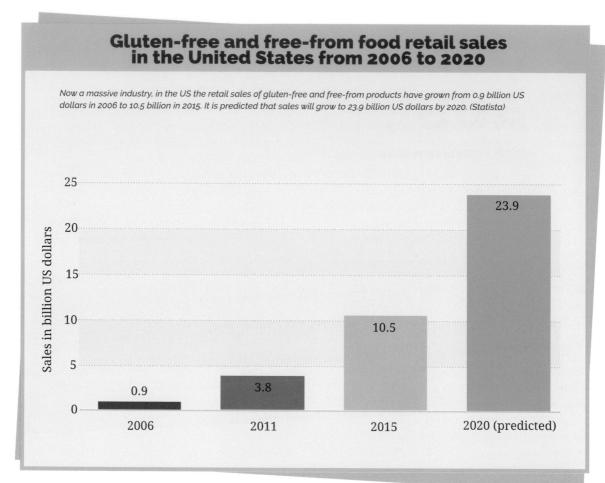

Gluten-free and free-from food retail sales in the United States from 2006 to 2020

Now a massive industry, in the US the retail sales of gluten-free and free-from products have grown from 0.9 billion US dollars in 2006 to 10.5 billion in 2015. It is predicted that sales will grow to 23.9 billion US dollars by 2020. (Statista)

Sales in billion US dollars

2006	0.9
2011	3.8
2015	10.5
2020 (predicted)	23.9

The bottom line: In the heat of the debate about the adverse effects of gluten, it is often forgotten that wheat and other cereals make a broad contribution to diets. For example, data from the UK National Diet and Nutrition Survey shows that bread alone contributes 11% of the nation's daily intake of protein, 18–21% of dietary fibre, 15–16% of iron and 15–19% of calcium. Wheat bran, found in wholegrain wheat, is rich in a range of what are known as phytochemicals, which help guard against coronary heart disease, stroke and cancer, and also aid digestion. Several studies have shown that gluten-free diets may be depleted in protein and nutrients compared to conventional diets, and that many people following gluten-free diets choose nutritionally inferior foods, such as gluten-free cakes and biscuits, rather than introducing healthier grains and pulses.

It is therefore an overreaction to assume that the health of more than a small proportion of the population will be improved by eliminating wheat or gluten from the diet. In fact, the opposite may occur if important nutrients provided by wheat are not replaced from an alternative source.

DOES LACTOSE CAUSE BLOATING?

Another condition that is popular among the self-diagnosis brigade is lactose intolerance. High-profile celebrities often credit their enviable figures and glowing good looks to giving up dairy (rather than airbrushing) and many of the rest of us follow suit in the hope of achieving the same results.

THE TREND FOR GIVING up lactose is interesting, as researchers have found that early Neolithic Europeans couldn't stomach their milk, according to the first direct examination of lactose intolerance in skeletons dating from 5840 to 5000 BC. Nevertheless, dairy farming persisted – most probably because, unlike stream water, milk was free from parasites and safer to drink. Dairy farming became widespread and this drove the rapid evolution of lactose tolerance. This means that, today, 90% of adult Northern Europeans and some people from Africa and the Middle East possess a gene that means their bodies are able to successfully process dairy into useful nutrients.

WHAT IS LACTOSE?

Lactose is the main carbohydrate (known as a disaccharide) present in dairy products. During infancy, lactose accounts for most of our dietary carbohydrates. The concentration of lactose in breast milk is 7.2mg/100ml (0.00007oz/fl oz), whereas in cow's milk it is only 4.7mg/100ml.

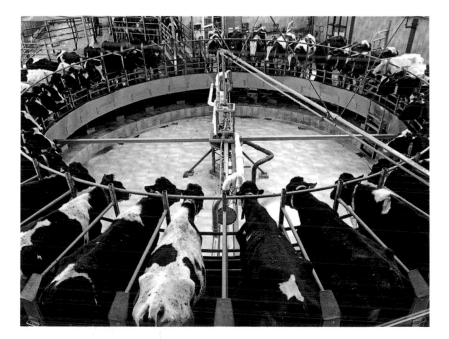

....

RIGHT: Dairy cattle are milked on average twice a day but may be milked up to five times a day.

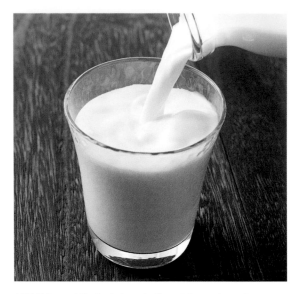

In order to be digested and absorbed, lactose requires the presence of the enzyme lactase in the small intestine. Levels of lactase production are at a peak for around the first six months after birth, and then decline to less than 10% of that level in childhood. However, lactase activity usually persists in populations where dairy products are consumed into adulthood. These are typically white Caucasians living in Northern and Western Europe and the USA.

TYPES OF LACTOSE INTOLERANCE

Lactose intolerance, which can also be called lactose malabsorption or hypolactasia, is caused by low lactase activity in the gut due to a deficiency in production. Lactose intolerance occurs when the lactose cannot be digested and absorbed and then causes symptoms.

Lactase deficiency has been described in three

ABOVE: A 250ml (8.5 fl.oz) glass of milk contains 12g (0.42 oz) of lactose.

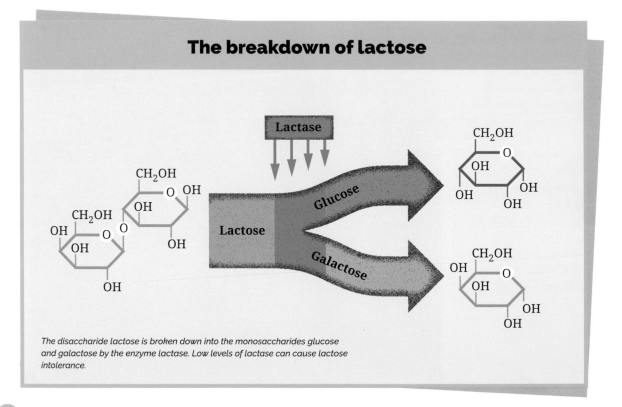

The breakdown of lactose

The disaccharide lactose is broken down into the monosaccharides glucose and galactose by the enzyme lactase. Low levels of lactase can cause lactose intolerance.

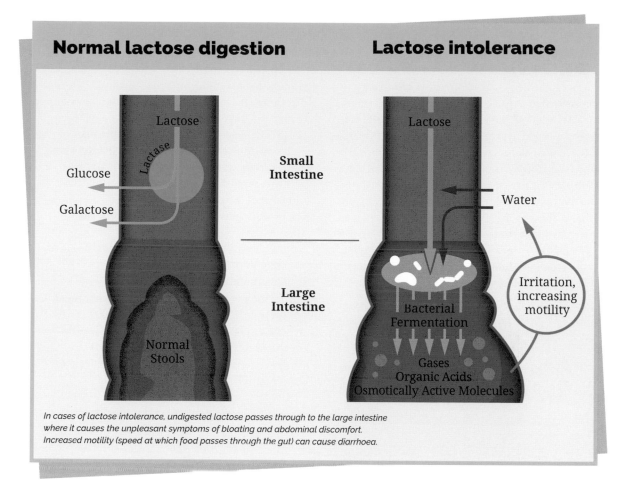

Normal lactose digestion

Lactose

Lactase

Glucose

Galactose

Small Intestine

Large Intestine

Normal Stools

Lactose intolerance

Lactose

Water

Bacterial Fermentation

Irritation, increasing motility

Gases
Organic Acids
Osmotically Active Molecules

In cases of lactose intolerance, undigested lactose passes through to the large intestine where it causes the unpleasant symptoms of bloating and abdominal discomfort. Increased motility (speed at which food passes through the gut) can cause diarrhoea.

different conditions: congenital, primary late onset and secondary onset. Congenital lactase deficiency is rare and symptoms occur shortly after birth. In the first year it is common for babies to experience partial malabsorption of lactose present in human milk or formula. This phenomenon of physiological malabsorption due to an insufficient production of the lactase enzyme may be the cause of colic. Insufficient lactase production generally only lasts for three months after birth, which coincides with the time that colicky behaviour usually subsides.

Primary late onset hypolactasia is a genetic condition that is characterized by a gradual reduction of lactase activity. Mostly, lactase deficiency manifests itself after the age of five in white populations and sometimes earlier in other racial groups. In some racial groups it does not occur before adolescence. Globally, it is the most common cause of lactose intolerance. In Europe, the frequency of primary late onset lactase deficiency varies from 2% in Scandinavia to 70% in some regions of Italy. The prevalence in the white population in the UK is about 20%. In Asia, the incidence is close to 100%.

Secondary hypolactasia is a shortage of lactase resulting from gastrointestinal disease causing damage to the lining of the small bowel. This damage may occur as a result of various conditions such as gastroenteritis, coeliac disease or inflammatory bowel disease (Crohn's disease).

Recovery of full function may take months, because lactase is the last enzyme to return to normal following injury. Clinically, secondary lactase deficiency occurs after small-bowel injury, such as viral and parasitic infections. Whether it makes sense to decrease lactose intake in infants with severe gastroenteritis for a limited period of time (one to three weeks) is heavily debated, not least because breast milk, which is recommended for infants, contains a high amount of lactose; the general consensus is that mothers should not stop breastfeeding because of gastroenteritis. Moreover, when lactose is fermented in the colon, it results in the growth of bifidobacteria, thus stimulating a healthy gut microbiota.

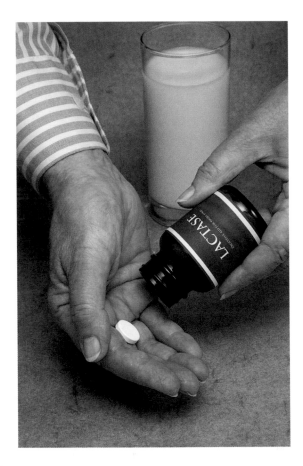

SYMPTOMS AND DIAGNOSIS

The presence of undigested lactose in the colon is responsible for fluid shifts that result in watery diarrhoea. Bacteria present in the colon ferment the lactose, resulting in the production of short-chain fatty acids, hydrogen, carbon dioxide and methane, which in turn cause bloating and cramps. Symptoms can increase with age, with many patients developing symptoms of lactose intolerance in adolescence and adulthood. They start shortly after consumption of milk and, although there are broad differences in response among patients, symptoms are in general related to the amount of lactose ingested.

If lactose intolerance is suspected, a true diagnosis can be made using a lactose hydrogen breath test. In exceptional circumstances, this may be confirmed by a duodenal biopsy. Other measures include examination of the pH of the faeces, a blood test and/or checking for the presence of lactose in the stool.

The lactose hydrogen breath test is a quick, non-invasive test that measures the content of hydrogen in expired air. A high level of hydrogen is indicative of undigested lactose. The lactose tolerance blood test measures levels of glucose in the blood after a challenge with lactose. Glucose is created when lactose breaks down. For this test, several blood samples need to be taken after the intake of milk.

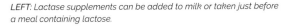

LEFT: Lactase supplements can be added to milk or taken just before a meal containing lactose.

TREATMENT

Treatment is via referral to a dietician, who will prescribe a lactose-free or lactose-poor diet. Completely lactose-free is only needed in the rare case of infants with congenital lactase deficiency. In all the other clinical situations, some lactase activity will persist, and thus "small" amounts of lactose can be tolerated. Indeed, most people with lactose intolerance will be able to consume up to 7g (0.25oz) of lactose (approximately 100ml/4fl oz of milk) without displaying symptoms. Some sufferers have even been shown to tolerate up to 500ml (20fl oz) of milk per day. Fermented dairy products such as cheese and yogurt are in general better tolerated, as the lactose is fermented by the probiotic strains added. In many countries, lactase can be administered as an "enzymatic supplement". This exists in both powder and liquid form, and needs to be taken just before a lactose-containing meal.

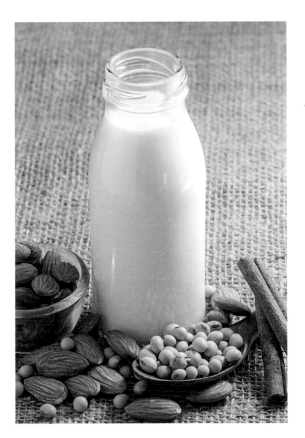

RIGHT: *Alternative milks such as soya and almond milks are lactose free and are usually fortified with calcium to match the amount in cow's milk.*

The bottom line: In the absence of a diagnosis of lactose intolerance it can be detrimental to health to avoid dairy products, as nutrition surveys show that they are important contributors to nutrient intakes. Dairy intakes are declining in populations who can tolerate them, potentially due to concerns regarding salt or saturated fat, but also for some as a misguided method for weight loss. This impacts on the intake of important nutrients such as protein, calcium, magnesium and B vitamins. Surveys show that dairy products provide over a third of the intake for calcium and vitamin B12.

Although there are an abundance of readily available non-milk alternatives to choose from, such as almond, soya, oat or rice milks, their nutrient profile is inferior compared with that of actual milk. Many of them also have added sugar. They contain much less protein than cow's milk and the plant protein is of a lower biological quality compared with that in cow's milk, meaning it lacks essential amino acids. They are generally not good sources of calcium, although most varieties have calcium added. However, the added calcium will not be as well absorbed as it would from cow's milk, due to the lack of protein, whose presence in cow's milk assists the absorption of calcium. Furthermore, dairy products have a low GI (glycaemic index), giving them the ability to satisfy, which is an important tool in maintaining a healthy weight.

DOES EVERYONE NEED PROBIOTICS?

The World Health Organization (WHO) defines probiotics as "live organisms which when administered in adequate amounts confer a health benefit on the host". "Probiotics" is a broad term for living microorganisms like bacteria and yeast.

THERE ARE THOUSANDS OF different types of probiotic bacteria, from lactobacilli (such as *Lactobacillus acidophilus* and *Lactobacillus rhamnosus GG*) to bifidobacteria (such as *Bifidobacterium bifidum*) and some yeasts (*Saccharomyces boulardii*). These organisms are similar to the ones already present in the digestive tract, so when you eat them – often in yogurts, or as food supplements – each strain can offer a different benefit to your body. But to influence the human gut microflora and provide a health benefit, probiotics must first survive the journey through the intestinal tract.

At present there are restrictions on the use of the term "probiotics" on food labelling and advertising, and instead you might see other terms such as "live bacteria". That's because use of the term "probiotic" is currently regarded as an unpermitted health claim: just because a label states that a product contains these live bacteria does not mean that the bacteria will be able to survive long enough to reach your gut or that the product contains enough bacteria to have a positive effect. And as there are several types of probiotics, with each strain thought to have different effects on the body, the term "probiotic" covers too many possibilities to guarantee health benefits.

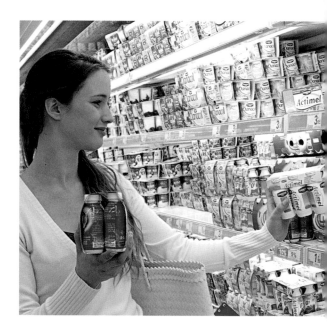

....

ABOVE: Products labelled as containing live bacteria may not have the same effects as those labelled as containing probiotic bacteria.

OPPOSITE ABOVE: Probiotic bacteria, shown here on small intestine tissue, are strains of bacteria that are able to survive through the acidic stomach into the lower intestine in adequate amounts to confer health benefits.

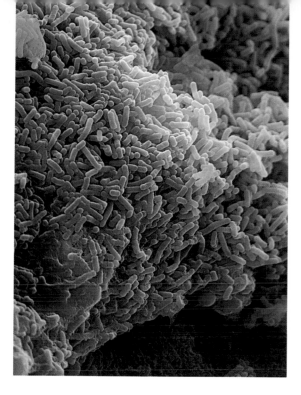

(*C. difficile*) infection. *C. difficile* is a potentially dangerous bacterium that can cause diarrhoea and life-threatening complications. It can infect the gut if the balance of bacteria is disturbed by antibiotic treatment.

Acute and infectious diarrhoea
Acute diarrhoea is common in infants and young children. It can have many causes, including bacterial or viral infections. There is some evidence that probiotics can slightly shorten the duration of diarrhoea caused by a stomach bug, by providing beneficial bacteria and therefore helping to restore a healthy balance of bacteria in the gut.

Irritable bowel syndrome (IBS)
IBS is a chronic condition characterized by abdominal pain, diarrhoea and/or constipation, and associated symptoms such as flatulence, bloating and urgency when needing the toilet. Research suggests that probiotics may help alleviate bloating and flatulence in some people with IBS. Again, this is due to the probiotics balancing the microflora in the gut. However, the full extent of the benefits is not known – and nor do we know the most effective probiotic strain. The UK's National Institute for Health and Care Excellence (NICE) guidelines on the diagnosis and management of IBS include advice on trying probiotics for at least four weeks while monitoring the effects.

Lactose intolerance
Some studies have found that certain probiotics such as *Lactobacillus acidophilus* may help reduce stomach cramps, flatulence and diarrhoea caused by lactose intolerance. However, research into this is still ongoing.

CONDITIONS WHERE PROBIOTICS CAN HELP
Antibiotic-associated diarrhoea (AAD)
There is good evidence that taking high doses of some probiotics (*Lactobacillus rhamnosus GG* or *Saccharomyces boulardii*) while taking antibiotics can reduce the risk of AAD. Antibiotics can sometimes strip out the protective bacteria in your gastrointestinal tract, leading to an imbalance in the microflora in the gut, which can cause diarrhoea. Probiotics can help by providing the beneficial bacteria and therefore restoring the correct balance of bacteria in the gut.

Probiotics consumed with antibiotics may also reduce the risk of developing a *Clostridium difficile*

The bottom line: Probiotics are thought to help restore the balance between good and bad bacteria in your gut when it has been disrupted by an illness or treatment.

If you are healthy, not on antibiotics, and not about to go into hospital or travel abroad, you probably don't need probiotics.

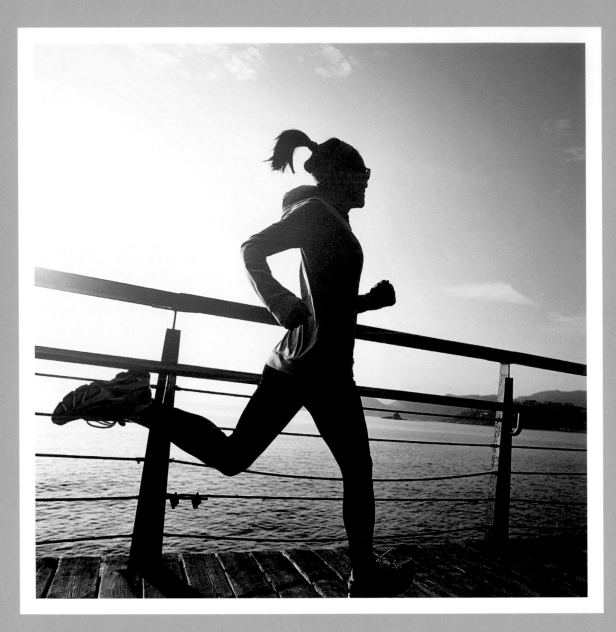

2

GIVE YOURSELF A BOOST

Myths relating to your metabolism

METABOLISM: AN OVERVIEW

Metabolism is a term covering all the chemical reactions that occur in the body that are necessary to maintain life. These metabolic processes include growth and repair, cell renewal and movement.

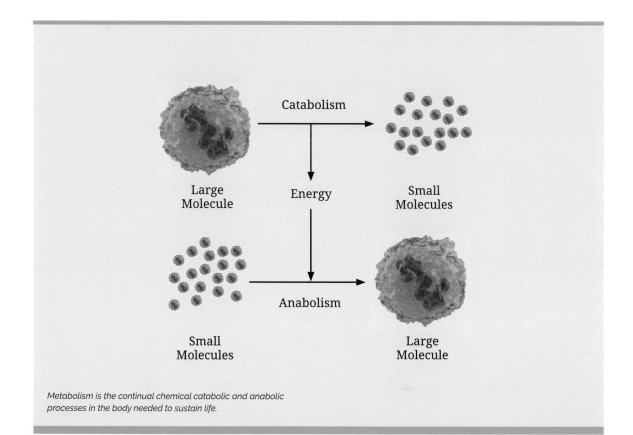

Metabolism is the continual chemical catabolic and anabolic processes in the body needed to sustain life.

AT ANY ONE TIME, there are millions of metabolic processes occurring simultaneously in our bodies. These processes can be divided into two groups. Anabolic processes use simple chemicals and molecules to manufacture a vast array of finished products – for example, the building of proteins from amino acids. On the other hand, catabolic processes break down complex molecules to release energy, which our bodies need – for example, the breakdown of starch into glucose.

The speed of these metabolic processes is commonly known as metabolic rate or energy expenditure and this determines the number of calories your body will use up in a given amount of time. The faster your metabolism, the more calories your body needs.

Metabolic rate can be divided into the following categories:

· Basal metabolic rate (BMR) is your metabolic rate when you are at deep rest, i.e. your digestive system is inactive and you have rested for at least eight hours. It is the amount of energy needed to control your temperature and breathing and to keep your heart, brain and nerves functioning.

· Resting metabolic rate (RMR) is often used interchangeably with BMR, but is measured using a different technique. It is the minimum metabolic rate required to keep you alive and functioning while not physically active. On average, it accounts for up to 50–75% of total calorie expenditure.

· Thermic effect of food (TEF) is the energy consumed when your body is digesting and processing food. When you eat, your metabolic rate rises. This rise represents approximately 10% of total energy expenditure.

· Thermic effect of exercise (TEE) is the energy consumed when you exercise.

· Non-exercise activity thermogenesis (NEAT) is the energy consumed during other activities. This includes everything from typing and hanging laundry to fidgeting.

....

BELOW: Specialist laboratory equipment can be used to accurately measure an individual's BMR.

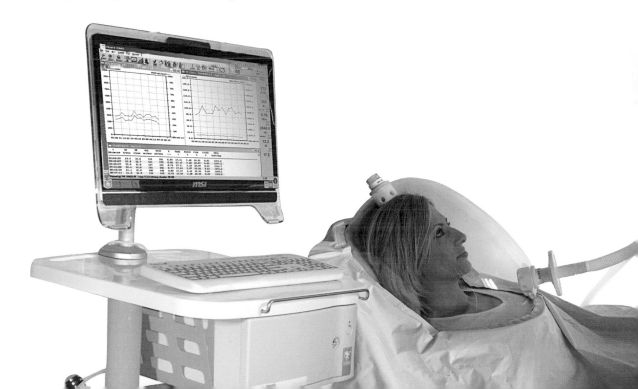

How to calculate your metabolic rate

For research purposes, metabolic rate can be measured by two methods:

- Direct calorimetry, which measures the subject's heat output through direct observation inside a calorimeter.
- Indirect calorimetry, which measures the heat output by using a calculation based on the difference between the amount of oxygen inhaled and the amount of carbon dioxide exhaled.

While man-sized calorimeters are not widely accessible, there are several handheld devices available to buy, but these can be very expensive and not completely accurate.

If you don't have a machine to hand, equations can be used to work out your BMR. The formula known as the Harris-Benedict equation was first developed in 1918 and over the years has been tweaked and updated to be more suited to our improved health status a century later.

BMR Calculation for Women:
(10 × weight in kg) + (6.25 × height in cm) – (5 × age in years) – 161

BMR Calculation for Men:
(10 × weight in kg) + (6.25 × height in cm) – (5 × age in years) + 5

To then find out your body's energy needs, you should factor in your daily activity and exercise level.

Level of Exercise	Daily Calories Needed
Little to no exercise	BMR x 1.2
Light exercise (1 to 3 days per week)	BMR x 1.4
Moderate exercise (3 to 5 days per week)	BMR x 1.6
Heavy exercise (6 to 7 days per week)	BMR x 1.8
Very heavy exercise (intense workouts twice a day)	BMR x 1.9

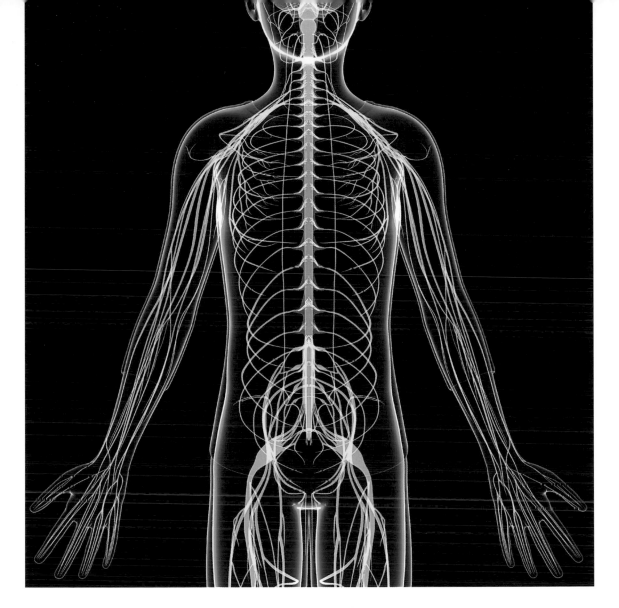

An individual's BMR will differ according to their body size (how tall they are and how much they weigh), their body composition (how much muscle they have in relation to fat) and their age. The bigger you are the more calories you need for basic functions. And the more muscle you have the more calories you use, even if those muscles are resting. Gender is also a factor and men have a higher basal metabolic rate than women because their muscle-to-fat ratio is generally higher than women's. This means that an average man will burn more calories than an average woman of the same age and weight.

....

ABOVE: BMR is the energy required to keep the complex web of nerves and neurons known as the nervous system functioning.

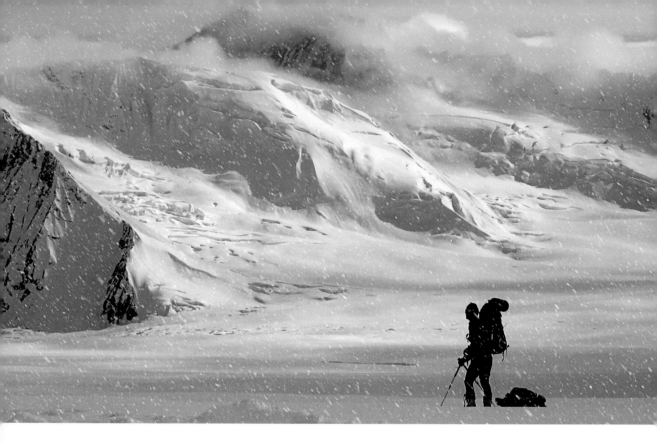

WHAT AFFECTS YOUR METABOLISM?

As we get older, changes in body composition, hormones and lifestyle result in a lower calorie requirement. With ageing, muscle mass drops, resulting in a higher fat-to-muscle ratio, and the natural decline in BMR means we need fewer calories. Hormone levels drop as we age, with men producing less testosterone and women producing less oestrogen, both of which are involved in anabolic processes that use up energy. It is particularly a problem for women approaching the menopause, as this brings with it a significant drop in hormones that normally promote energy use. Many women find it harder to lose weight during this time.

Other factors that can influence metabolic rate include environmental temperature and physical activity. When your body is exposed to cold, it needs to burn more calories to prevent its temperature from falling. Most people think that it is the amount of exercise you do that will have the biggest impact on

energy expenditure, but for most people this might actually only account for 5–10% of total expenditure, whereas NEAT (energy consumed through non-exercise activity) could account for as much as 30%.

Genetics influence metabolism too, which means that metabolic rates do vary between individuals from birth. However, experts disagree on just how much these genetic differences can actually account for variations in weight, as there are so many more factors that can have a much larger impact. It is a common belief that slim people have a faster metabolism and overweight people have a slower metabolism, but this is very rarely the case. Despite the common belief that metabolism determines whether someone is fat or thin, weight gain is primarily due to energy imbalance – taking on more calories than you expend.

ABOVE: Climate influences metabolic rate; the colder the temperature the faster a person's metabolic rate will be.

What affects your BMR?

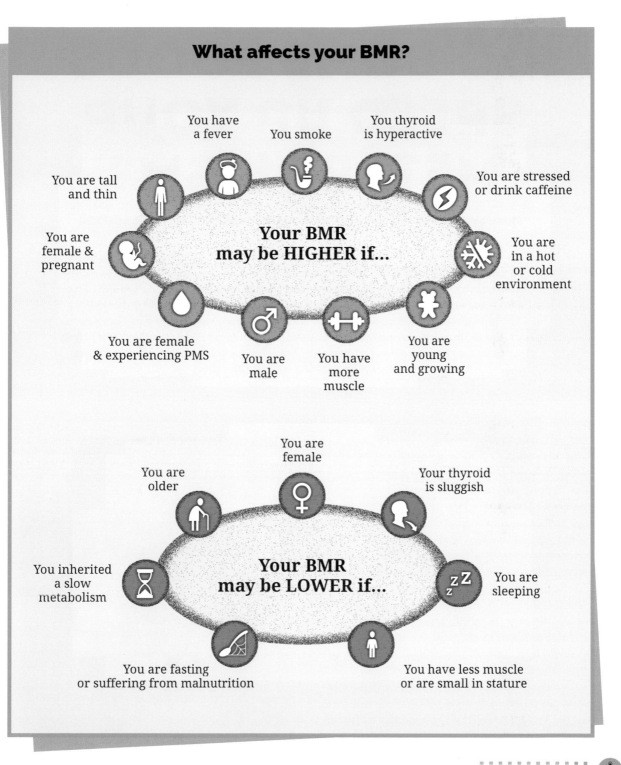

You have a fever

You smoke

You thyroid is hyperactive

You are tall and thin

You are stressed or drink caffeine

Your BMR may be HIGHER if...

You are female & pregnant

You are in a hot or cold environment

You are female & experiencing PMS

You are male

You have more muscle

You are young and growing

You are female

You are older

Your thyroid is sluggish

You inherited a slow metabolism

Your BMR may be LOWER if...

You are sleeping

You are fasting or suffering from malnutrition

You have less muscle or are small in stature

DO SOME FOODS SPEED UP YOUR METABOLISM?

As we have learned, the thermic effect of food (TEF) is the energy consumed when your body is digesting and processing food. It can, to a small extent, be influenced by the composition of our diet and the types of foods we eat. The primary determinants of daily TEF are the total caloric content of our meals and their macronutrient composition, whereas meal frequency has little to no effect. It has been claimed that, in obese individuals, TEF is reduced, meaning they miss out on the effect of burning calories to offset intake, but to date research has failed to validate this.

THE THERMIC EFFECT of protein is the highest, with 20 to 35% of the energy provided by protein being required for its digestion and absorption. The thermic effect of carbohydrates averages between 15 and 20% of the calories in those foods and will depend on whether they are simple sugars or complex starches, as well as the amount of fibre present. Most easily digested are fats, which have a thermic effect of only 5%. This means that your net caloric gain from fats averages 95% of their total calories, compared with a net caloric gain of about 70% of the calories in lean protein.

Some foods, such as celery, are often claimed to have negative calories (requiring more energy to digest than is recovered from the food), but there is no evidence to support this hypothesis. One recent study from Oxford Brookes University investigated the thermic effects of chilli and coconut oil (which contain a type of fat known as medium-chain

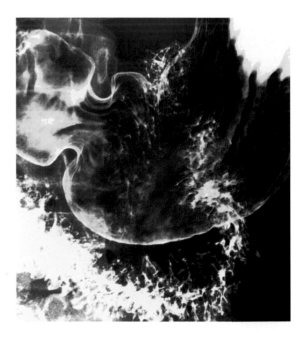

TRUST ME, I'M A DIETICIAN

How to speed up your metabolism

While some people turn to certain food and drinks in the hope of speeding up their metabolism, others are resigned to the belief that there is nothing they can do and that they have just been dealt an unlucky genetic hand. While there are certain factors you can't change, such as your age or your height, you can change your body composition by building more muscle, and this in turn will speed up your basal metabolic rate. Muscle tissue burns more calories than fat tissue, so increasing your muscle mass will help you lose weight. Two sessions of muscle-strengthening exercise per week should be sufficient to achieve results. The exercise should work all major muscle groups (legs, hips, back, abdomen, chest, shoulders and arms) – for instance lifting weights and high-intensity interval training (HIIT) workouts.

Aerobic activity will also speed up metabolism, not only through the calories burned while you are exercising but also through the effect of the afterburn, when the body

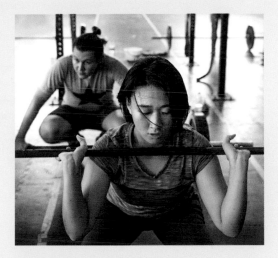

continues to burn calories for a number of hours after the exercise has stopped.

Some people who are said to have a fast metabolism are probably just more fidgety than others. As NEAT can account for such a major chunk of calories burned, it pays to be constantly busy.

triglycerides, MCT). The researchers concluded that adding chilli and MCT to meals increases TEF by over 50%, which over time may accumulate to help induce weight loss and prevent weight gain (see also page 121).

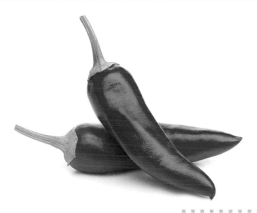

OPPOSITE: An X-ray of a healthy human stomach.

RIGHT: A recent study found that adding chilli to food increases its thermic effect.

DOES DIETING RUIN METABOLISM?

A common complaint of people who struggle to lose weight is that previous dieting has ruined their metabolism. Metabolic adaptation, also known as adaptive thermogenesis or starvation mode, may be an influencing factor in the development of obesity but it is not solely responsible and can be overcome with sufficient dietary change and exercise. Such change may require more effort, commitment and determination than the failed dieter has bargained for.

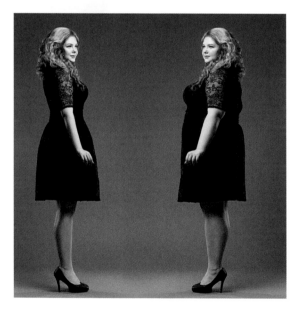

ABOVE: Previous crash dieting cannot be blamed for subsequent weight gain.

IN RESPONSE TO STARVATION, metabolic rate slows to compensate for the calorie deficit. The extent to which metabolic rate decreases during calorie restriction and weight loss is highly variable between individuals.

Most studies show that obese people have a higher total and resting metabolic rate compared to normal-weight individuals, because it takes more energy to move a bigger body. They also have more tissue, both muscle and fat, which is metabolically active to different degrees. Interestingly, studies show that people who have previously been overweight or obese and then lost weight to reach a healthy level have a metabolic rate that is 3–8% lower than those who have never been overweight; other studies show that, as people gain weight, their metabolic rate increases proportionally. This means it may be slightly harder for previously obese people to maintain their new healthy weight, but this is something that can be overcome with a bit of extra exercise.

The bottom line: While it may be the case that weight maintenance is challenging, the metabolism is never ruined. A lower metabolic rate can be overcome with additional exercise that helps to build muscle mass.

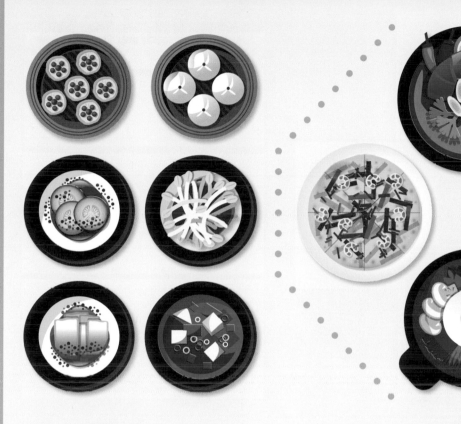

Some people believe that eating six small meals a day, and splitting your daily calories into smaller groups, is better than eating the traditional three. This is linked to the knowledge that each time you eat there is a rise in metabolic rate through the thermic effect of food. However, there is very little evidence that breaking up meals this way leads to an increase in net metabolic rate. This is because the thermic effect of food is directly proportionate to the energy consumed in a meal. The foods you eat in one sitting or in two will have the same effect on your metabolism.

There is, though, some evidence to suggest that how you consume your calories may impact on other aspects of your health. In one small study, 11 obese women were divided into two groups. They all consumed the same number of calories a day, but one group consumed these in two meals and the other in six meals. Both groups lost around the same amount of weight, but those who ate six meals retained more muscle mass whereas those who ate two meals had improved levels of cholesterol and better blood-sugar control.

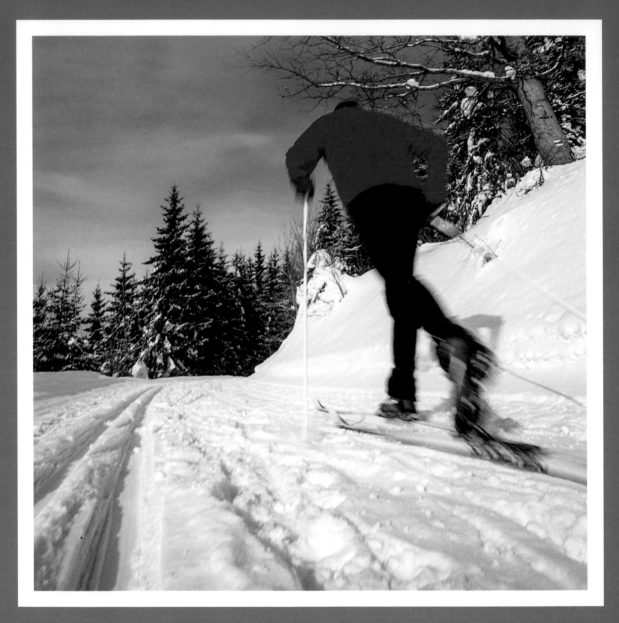

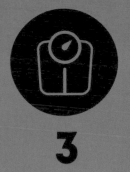

3

ALL ABOUT BALANCE

Myths relating to energy

ENERGY BALANCE: AN OVERVIEW

Energy balance is the relationship between energy in (energy taken into the body through food and drink) and energy out (energy being used in the body).

THIS RELATIONSHIP IS UNDERPINNED by the first law of thermodynamics, which states that energy cannot be created or destroyed but instead changes from one form to another. In other words, we may convert the energy stored in food into heat or we may store it as fat. The energy balance dictates whether weight is lost, gained or remains the same.

Energy is provided by the carbohydrate, protein and fat in the food and drinks we consume. It is also provided by alcohol. Depending on their composition, different food and drinks provide different amounts of energy.

Energy is measured in units of kilocalories (kcal) or kilojoules (kJ), with 1kcal being equal to 4.18kJ.

- Fat contains 9kcal (37kJ) per gram (25g = 1oz)
- Alcohol contains 7kcal (29kJ) per gram
- Protein contains 4kcal (17kJ) per gram
- Carbohydrate contains 3.75kcal (16kJ) per gram

On the flip side, different activities use up different amounts of calories. Strenuous activities such as running and heavy gardening use up more than reading or driving. Cross-country skiing is often billed as one of the most energetic activities, probably from a combination of the effort involved and the fact that it is performed in a cold environment, which means the body has to use up more energy to maintain its core temperature.

Because this balance of calories consumed in food and expended in exercise is common knowledge, calorie-tracking has become very popular. Sophisticated gadgets track your movements throughout the day and will estimate your total energy expenditure based on personal details such as your age and weight. You can then input details of your diet to see if your energy intake is a near match for your expenditure.

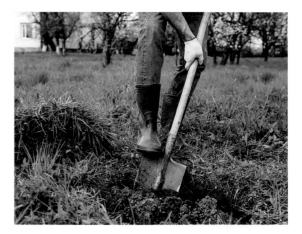

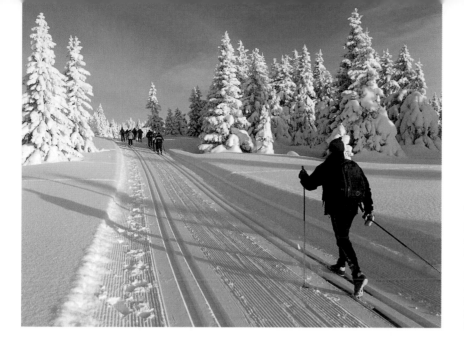

LEFT: Cross-country skiing is considered one of the highest calorie-burning activities.

OPPOSITE BELOW: Although not perceived as formal exercise, gardening can burn as many calories as a workout in the gym.

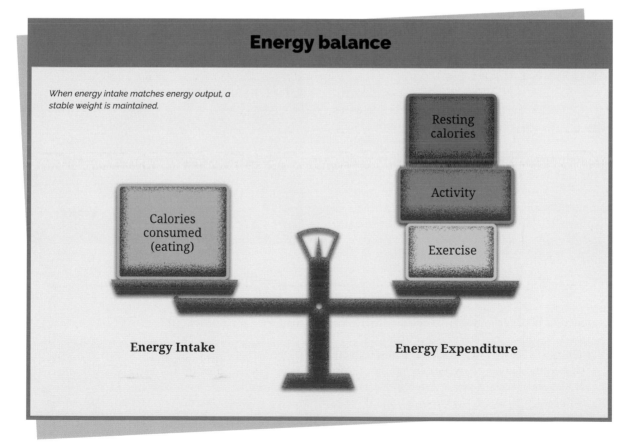

Energy balance

When energy intake matches energy output, a stable weight is maintained.

Resting calories

Activity

Calories consumed (eating)

Exercise

Energy Intake

Energy Expenditure

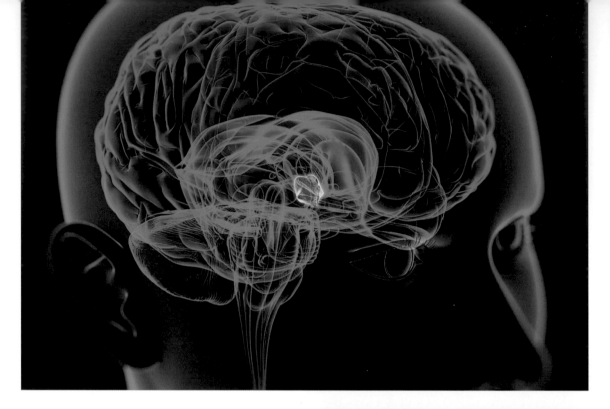

STAYING BALANCED

Since we can keep tabs on our diets using gadgets, you'd think that maintaining energy balance would be simple. But in reality it is regulated by a complex network of systems involving the hypothalamus (a part of the brain that controls many functions of the nervous and endocrine systems), nerves and hormones. Information is gathered about energy repletion/depletion, physical activity level, the stage of reproductive cycle or developmental state (such as pregnancy), as well as the types and amounts of foods eaten. This information influences the processes that affect energy balance.

This means the body is highly adaptable to a variety of energy intakes and outputs. It has to be adaptable in order to survive, and so mechanisms are in place to ensure stable energy transfer regardless of any energy imbalances. For example, a severe negative energy balance can lead to a decline in metabolism. When the body detects an energy deficit, it begins to slow down all functions that aren't essential for survival.

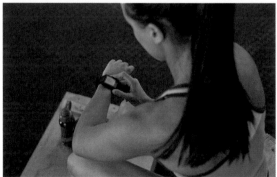

TOP: The hypothalamus is a small portion of the brain; one of its most important jobs is to link the functions of nerves and hormones.

ABOVE: Devices that measure your activity level are growing in popularity.

Both sides of the energy balance equation are complex and it is the relationship between energy intake and energy expenditure that will determine body composition and health outcomes.

Energy and survival

The next time you hear someone say "I've got no energy", you could in fact point out that as long as they drink water, they probably have enough stored energy to last for three to six weeks (maybe say it silently if you wish to remain friends). The amount of time a person can survive without food depends on factors such as body weight, genes and health status. Most importantly it depends on hydration, as in the absence of water death may occur after 24–72 hours.

Unlike total starvation, a person may survive semi-starvation for many months, or even years. This has been documented by survivors of famine and concentration and prisoner-of-war camps. During this time the body is able to moderate metabolism to conserve energy, although survival rates will differ between individuals and will be influenced by quality of food eaten and intake of the nutrients provided, which can cause or worsen disease through the development of deficiencies. The body's ability to alter its metabolism occurs through changes in thyroid function and over time a shift in the genetic make-up of certain races has evolved to enable them to survive long periods of semi-starvation, such as regular famine, through the better economical use of energy. The persistence of these genes in an obesogenic environment (availability to abundance of high-fat and -sugar foods and low levels of physical activity) is a root cause of the increased prevalence of diabetes in these racial groups.

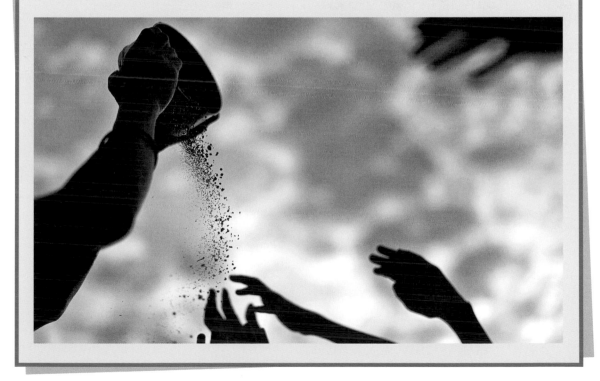

ARE ALL CALORIES CREATED EQUAL?

High-protein, low-carb diets have gained in popularity as they achieve the best weight-loss results. Initially, such diets were rejected by nutrition experts and dieticians in favour of the conventional low-fat, high-starch approach.

IF YOU DO THE MATHS, low-fat diets should have a lower calorie content as fat has more calories than carbohydrate and high-protein diets usually contain more fat. However, the principle of high-protein, low-carb diets has now gained some acceptance among academics, and sparked a huge debate. Could it be that calories from particular types of food affect the body differently?

A calorie, by its simplest definition, is a unit of energy. In the popular press and in the labelling of food products, a food calorie actually refers to a kilocalorie, or 1,000 calories. That is, 1 food cal equals 1kcal. According to thermodynamics,

energy can neither be created nor destroyed, so a calorie is of course a calorie. How is it possible, then, that calories from different nutrients produce different results?

METABOLIZABLE ENERGY

There are a number of factors that influence the impact of different types of food on the energy available to the body. When energy from the combustion of food is measured in experimental conditions in a test tube, it is known as absolute energy, but the energy actually available to the body after the food has been eaten is known as the metabolizable energy. The two amounts are unlikely to be the same, because not all of that food will be digested and absorbed – some will be lost from the body in urine and faeces.

Of the three energy-providing nutrients – namely protein, carbohydrate and fat – it is protein that has the highest absolute energy compared with metabolizable energy. This is because a number of the products of protein breakdown are used by the body for the excretion of excess nitrogen; these substances can account for up to 23% of the total energy of the food. The energy available from different protein foods depends on the chemical structure of the protein; more energy is lost from the consumption of meat protein compared with vegetable protein.

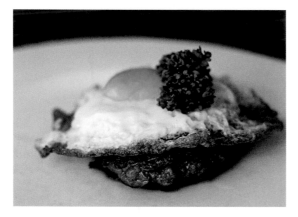

ABOVE: High-protein, low-carbohydrate diets have replaced low-fat diets in the quest for weight loss.

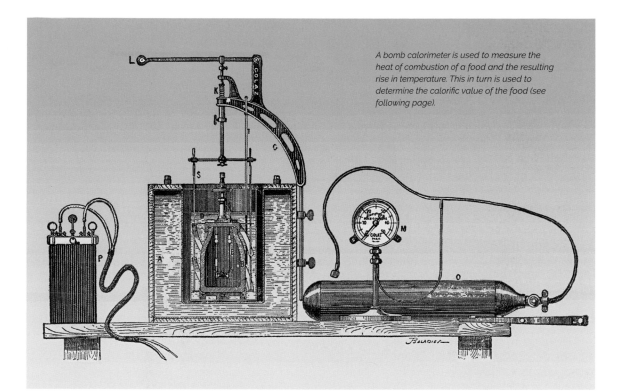

A bomb calorimeter is used to measure the heat of combustion of a food and the resulting rise in temperature. This in turn is used to determine the calorific value of the food (see following page).

How filling is your food?

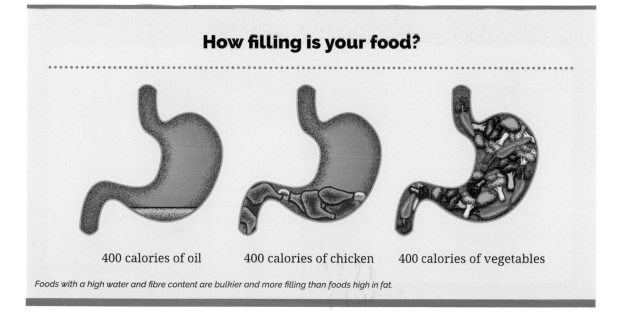

400 calories of oil   400 calories of chicken   400 calories of vegetables

Foods with a high water and fibre content are bulkier and more filling than foods high in fat.

ATWATER FACTORS

At the end of the nineteenth century, the scientist Wilbur Atwater devised "coefficients of availability" for protein, carbohydrate and fat. These are derived from the heats of combustion of protein, fat and carbohydrate, corrected for losses in digestion, absorption and excretion of nitrogenous waste products. For his experiments Atwater used foods that were typical of the American diet at that time, such as beef, butter, biscuits and baked beans, and calculated a single value for each of the energy-providing nutrients, regardless of which food it was contained within. These values are 4 calories per gram for protein, 9 calories per gram for fat and 4 calories per gram for carbohydrate (25g = 1oz). These so-called Atwater factors are still used today to assess the energy value of a single food.

THE FIBRE FACTOR

In the early 1970s it was recognized that separate factors were needed to take into account the division of total carbohydrate into available carbohydrate and fibre. Available carbohydrate was given a new value of 3.75 calories per gram. More recent research has shown large differences in the digestibility of foods, which are not accounted for by the Atwater factors. A classic example of this is almonds: studies have shown that about 20% of the calories in almonds are not available for digestion or absorption because of the nut's fibrous cell walls. Nuts are often rejected as too calorific by people wishing to lower their calorie intake, yet their low digestibility

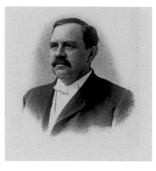

RIGHT: Chemist Wilbur Olin Atwater (1844–1907).

BELOW: The cellular structure of almonds means that not all their calories can be digested.

is a significant reason (among others) that the daily inclusion of a handful of nuts can actually help with weight loss. Consuming more dietary fibre results in the excretion not just of the fibre but also of fat and nitrogenous substances, which have an energy value, and it decreases the amount of time it takes for foods to pass through the digestive system. This "decreased transit time" gives food less of an opportunity to be fully digested and absorbed, so more is lost in the faeces. This means that applying the Atwater factors to a high-fibre diet could overestimate the

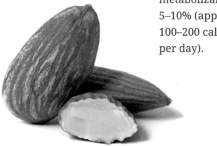

metabolizable energy by 5–10% (approximately 100–200 calories per day).

The bottom line: Differences in the energy lost during metabolism and fermentation can also influence the weight-loss effects of our diets. A greater amount of energy is used to fuel metabolism of protein, for example, while some of the energy in fermentable carbohydrate is lost through the production of gas. This may explain why weight loss is greater on a high-protein, high-fibre diet compared with a different diet of equal calories.

Of course, the increased energy expenditure associated with increased protein intake still does not violate the laws of thermodynamics. It does, however, suggest that diets that induce a difference in energy expenditure can introduce a difference in energy balance and thus a difference in weight loss.

IS THE 3,500-CALORIE RULE FOOLPROOF?

Before the popularity of celebrity magazines, newsagents' shelves were dominated by "slimming" magazines and diets that calculated different ways to cut 3,500 calories – the energy content of one pound of body fat.

AND IT WASN'T JUST the magazines that used this formula: for many years it was widely accepted within the medical profession and patients were told that if they could cut 500 calories per day from their diets (3,500 per week) they could lose a pound of fat each week. However, as many would-be dieters have discovered, it might work for the first week, and even the second and third, if you have a lot of weight to lose, but eventually this formula stops working and weight loss frustratingly plateaus.

LOSING MUSCLE MASS

The 3,500-calorie rule is based on a calculation made by researcher Max Wishnofsky in 1958, who concluded that 1lb (454g) of fat stores approximately 3,500kcal of energy.

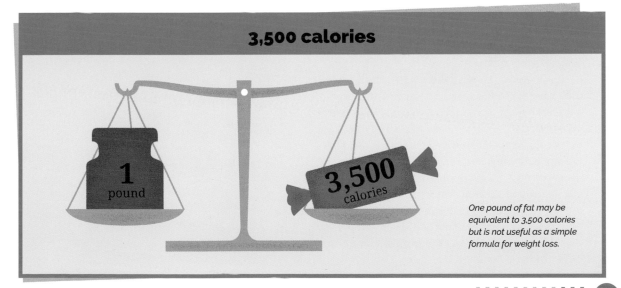

3,500 calories

1 pound

3,500 calories

One pound of fat may be equivalent to 3,500 calories but is not useful as a simple formula for weight loss.

However, when a person starts to lose weight they won't just lose fat; they will also lose lean body mass, mostly as muscle. Muscle mass can be preserved with the right type of exercise and by maintaining an adequate protein intake, but this will differ from person to person, making the 3,500-calorie rule inaccurate. As you lose weight, your BMR (basal metabolic rate) drops and the calorie deficit is harder to maintain (unless you restrict your calories more or exercise more). For example, if your body needed 2,600 calories a day to be in energy balance and you reduced your intake by 500 calories to 2,100, you would lose weight. But once you'd lost 20% of your weight, your body would only need 2,200 calories a day to stay in energy balance, so if you continued to eat 2,100 calories, your weight loss would stall.

CALCULATING THE DEFICIT

In addition to this, the longer you diet the more efficient your body becomes, as it makes metabolic adjustments in order to cope with the fact that it is receiving less food. Taking into account these factors, new, more sophisticated weight-loss models have been developed. They calculate the number of calories needed to maintain energy balance based on an individual's baseline data – that is, their age, gender, size and body composition – and predict the calorie deficit required to continue to lose weight over time as some of the parameters change.

These models show that the 3,500-calorie rule is only valid (at best) for the first month after starting a diet. However, it should be remembered that the early rapid weight-loss phase will mainly be thanks to loss of glycogen and water mass – not fat. This is not a bad thing; it's just how weight loss starts because when we reduce our calorie consumption, particularly of carbohydrates, our body feeds off the store of glycogen in our muscle tissue and liver. Glycogen is a mixture of carbohydrate and mostly water, so the first week of dieting always has the most dramatic result on the scales.

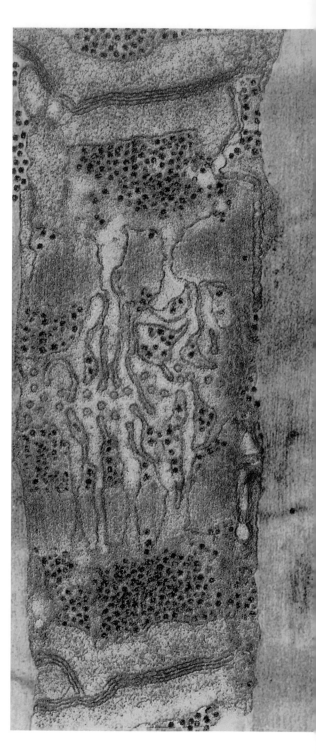

DO DIETS WORK?

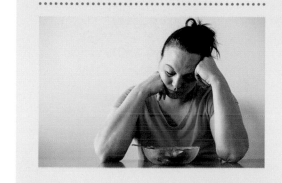

Overall, the body tries to prevent excessive swings of either positive or negative energy but for those who want to lose weight this is often interpreted as diets not working. With a restriction of calories comes a decline in metabolic rate, but if the energy deficit is high enough, the decline in metabolic rate will not be enough to negate it, and consequently both muscle and fat will be lost. However, the loss of muscle will further decrease metabolic rate and cause weight loss to slow to such an extent that the results become unnoticeable, at which point many dieters lose motivation and give up.

Diets do work but they work much better in conjunction with exercise, especially resistance exercise that will maintain muscle mass.

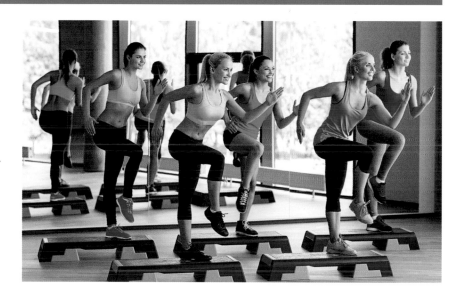

OPPOSITE: Glycogen is a polysaccharide that is the main form of storage of glucose in body tissues.

RIGHT: Exercise is important for weight loss, but is unlikely to succeed without calorie restriction.

The bottom line: So what should you do if the 3,500-calorie rule stops working? You can aim to maintain a 20% calorie deficit through a combination of increased exercise and cutting calorie intake, but this relies on having a fairly accurate measure of your daily calorie expenditure. Alternatively you can just keep your daily total of calories very low: 1,200 for a woman and 1,400 for a man. Research seems to suggest that calorie restriction is best for achieving weight loss, and exercise is more important for maintenance.

CAN YOU TARGET FAT LOSS?

Some diets come with the promise of making you drop a dress size, while some exercise routines claim to be able to eliminate bingo wings or achieve a flat tummy. Targeted fat loss, also known as spot-reduction, is a popular idea because most of us have parts of our bodies we like and bits we don't.

ALTHOUGH IT SEEMS LOGICAL that exercising a certain body part, such as the tops of the arms or the stomach muscles, should use up the fat in that area, it doesn't work like this. The fat contained in fat cells exists in a form known as triglycerides, which working muscle cells cannot use. It must be broken down into free fatty acids, which then enter the bloodstream. As a result, the fat broken down to be used as fuel during prolonged exercise can come from anywhere in your body, not just the part that is being worked the most.

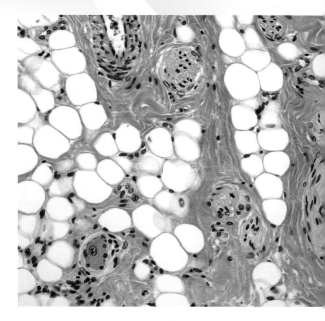

RIGHT: Adipose tissue (body fat) is made up mainly of adipocytes, specialized cells designed to store varying sizes of fat droplets, some of which can be very large.

The bottom line: The claim that a diet or a certain combination of foods can target fat loss from the desired area is sheer nonsense. It is impossible to predict exactly where weight will be lost, and patterns of weight loss vary greatly from one person to the next. Your genes influence fat distribution in the body, where you store it most and from where you will lose it. It is likely that, if you have recently gained weight in a certain area, such as around the stomach, this is the area from which you will first lose it when you start to diet, but tricky areas such as tops of arms and love handles, which are relatively small pockets of fat, are likely to remain, even if you are at your ideal weight.

TRUST ME, I'M A DIETICIAN

Targeting bingo wings

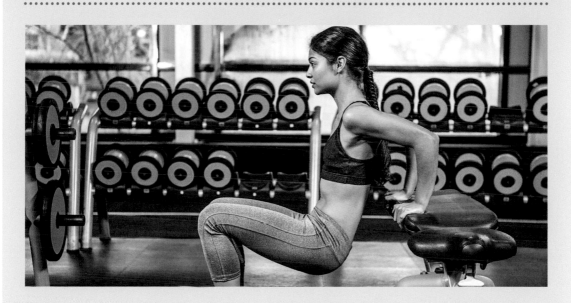

Women's arms are a constant source of fascination for the tabloid press. Even celebrity royals like Madonna and Michelle Obama have been caught out by the unflattering angle of the paparazzi's long lenses. Bingo wings are little pockets of stubborn fat at the tops of the arms; they wobble when you clap your hands and you can pinch the fat away from the muscle.

Although bingo wings are difficult to get rid of, it is not impossible. But it is not a case of converting fat into muscle. It is a popular myth that you can turn fat into muscle with the right exercise or that muscle will turn to fat if you don't work out. Only a combination of diet and targeted exercise can help to reduce the appearance of bingo wings. There are no

particular foods that will have a magical effect on your arms alone. Rather, it is a case of eating less to create a calorie deficit that will allow fat stores to be mobilized and used as energy. Fat will be lost from all over the body, and you may not notice much of an impact on your arms at first, but eventually some fat will be lost here.

Exercising the triceps muscles (behind the biceps) will tone and strengthen your arms, giving them a sleeker appearance. Exercises for the triceps muscles include closed-hand push-ups, bench dips and triceps pushbacks. For best results aim to do a 10-to-15-minute workout every other day. Be warned, don't expect an instantaneous change; it may take 8 to 12 weeks to see results.

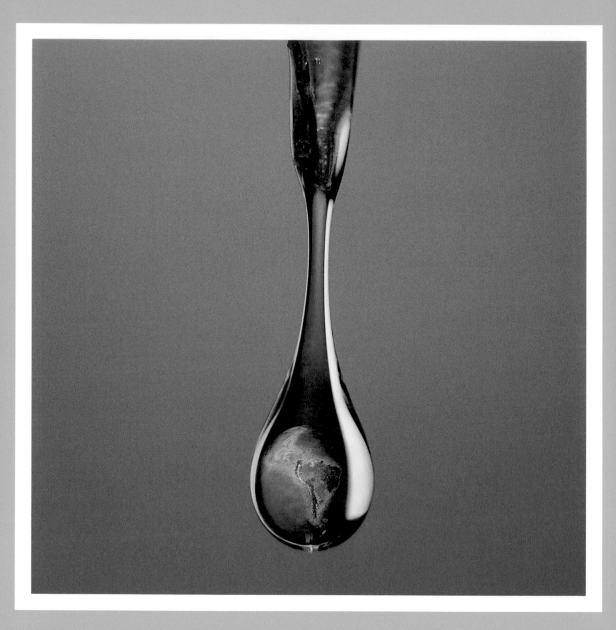

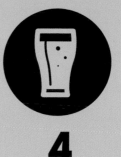

4

STAYING HYDRATED

Myths relating to water consumption,
thirst and dehydrating drinks

HYDRATION: AN OVERVIEW

Since the 1980s, there has been a shift in society's attitude to drinking water. Rather than simply turning on the tap, consumers now prefer to buy bottled, canned, carbonated or flavoured water, water with added or removed ingredients such as vitamins, trace elements or herbal extracts, or even water with ingredients removed, such as sodium.

DRINKING BOTTLED WATER IS in vogue, with some restaurants offering water from detached icebergs, tropical islands or mountainous regions. Water menus now sit comfortably alongside wine, whisky and cocktail menus in their descriptions of taste, flavour, origin, history and price. Indeed, water and hydration status are increasingly recognized by consumers as being an important part of a healthy lifestyle, as well as of sports and exercise regimes. In scientific studies, drinking water has been associated with better diets and healthier behaviours. But how much water do we actually need and, in the absence of bottled water, will tap (plain) water suffice?

It is a given that water is the most abundant substance on our planet, but it is also the most abundant substance in our bodies. Water is an essential transporter: in the form of blood, it transports "good" substances around the body (e.g. hormones and nutrients) and removes "bad" substances such as toxins and waste products to the liver and kidneys for clearance. Water is essential for helping us regulate body temperature and prevents us from overheating during exercise. It also helps lubricate joints and organs such as the eyes. Around three quarters of an infant's body is composed of water, a value that decreases to two thirds by the time we reach adulthood. With our bodies so reliant on water, it makes sense that maintaining a balanced hydration level is crucial. But what is the best way to strike that balance – and do other fluids count towards hydration?

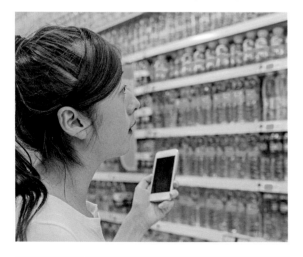

ABOVE: We have more types of water to choose from than ever before.

SOURCES OF WATER

Over the years, many scientific groups have assessed the evidence to establish recommendations for total water intake. Typically the amount recommended per day from ALL sources – and I'll elaborate on this shortly – is around 2 litres (4 pints) for adolescent and adult females and 2.5 litres (5 pints) for adolescent and adult males. Lower values are recommended for younger ages. However, requirements can increase with exercise, in hot environments and in certain life stages such as pregnancy and breastfeeding. In general, total body water tends to be higher if you are male, and have increased muscularity and reduced amounts of fat, so recommended intakes are factored accordingly.

All scientific recommendations point to water intake being the best way to stay hydrated, whether it is from the tap or bottle, but other beverages and liquids such as teas, coffees, milks, "soft" drinks, juices and soups contribute too. Water also counts if it comes from food. The water content of cow's milk is >90%, with fruit and vegetables >80%, and hot meals ranging from 40% for a dish like lasagne to 70% for a vegetable stew. Only strong alcoholic drinks, such as wine and spirits, and bakery products (<40% water) do not rate. The water in a weak lager or shandy will count to begin with (from the first pint or half pint), but as more alcohol is drunk, the net loss of water overtakes the amount consumed. In terms of fluid intake, it is estimated that about 20% of our daily water (fluid) intake comes from food, and so, in simple terms, the remainder to be consumed from beverages may be loosely translated as around 8–10 x 200ml glasses, or 1.6–2 litres a day (around 3 to 4 pints).

BELOW: Percentage of body water decreases with age.

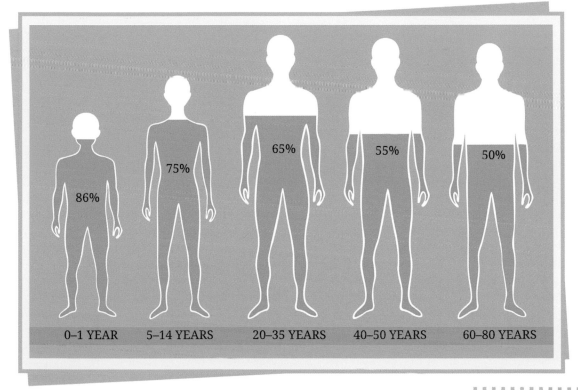

86% 0–1 YEAR
75% 5–14 YEARS
65% 20–35 YEARS
55% 40–50 YEARS
50% 60–80 YEARS

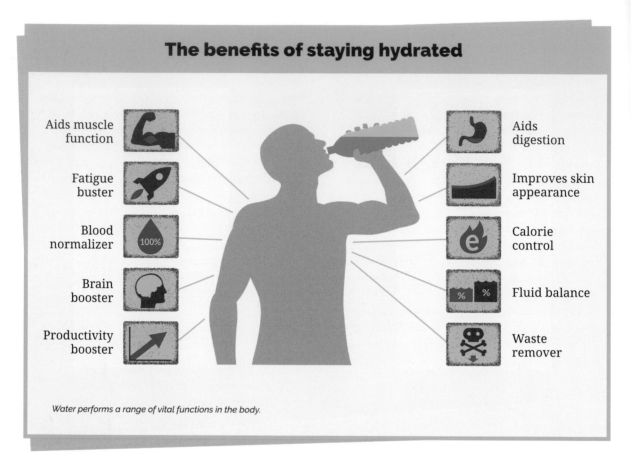

The benefits of staying hydrated

Aids muscle function

Fatigue buster

Blood normalizer

Brain booster

Productivity booster

Aids digestion

Improves skin appearance

Calorie control

Fluid balance

Waste remover

Water performs a range of vital functions in the body.

YOUR DRINK OF CHOICE

There's lots of choice in our supermarkets for satisfying this "8–10 glasses a day" guideline, with water and milk usually proposed as preferred options in terms of dental health and body-weight control. However, tea is the second most commonly consumed beverage in the world after water, while in the US the most popular hot drink is coffee. We choose our beverages based on individual preferences, taste, cost, and social and cultural norms and habits; for some people, considerations also include the presence or absence of sugars, vitamins, minerals, non-nutritive ingredients and sweeteners. All beverages can help hydrate but, as with most food guidance, there are caveats. For example, while sugar-sweetened beverages will contribute to hydration status, they can have a negative impact on dental health and overall energy intakes. Diet drinks have none of the calories but contain phosphoric acid, which can, following frequent consumption and/or high intake, trigger dental erosion. Similarly, although fruit juices and smoothies can contribute to hydration while also providing vitamins and minerals, they can be acidic in nature and contain sugar, which can be harmful to dental health. Any more than 150ml (5fl oz) of juice per day provides good amounts of some vitamins but overdoes the free sugars.

And so back to bottled water: does it make a difference if water is bottled or not, carbonated, filtered or cleansed using reverse-osmosis deionizing filters? In terms of hydration, the answer is "no": tap water will be just as effective. After that, it is a matter of consumer choice.

IF YOU'RE THIRSTY, ARE YOU DEFINITELY DEHYDRATED?

It could be argued that the sensation of thirst is one of the most essential biological stimuli. The instinct of thirst is believed to have been responsible for the successful colonization by vertebrates of dry land.

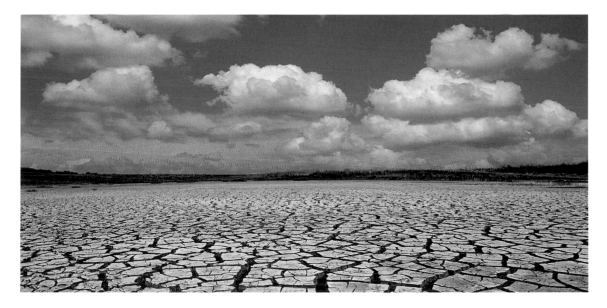

HUMANS CAN'T TYPICALLY SURVIVE for more than three days without water. So recognizing one is thirsty – and responding to it – is essential for life.

Thirst and our responses to it remain to be fully understood, with functional magnetic resonance imaging (MRI) scans suggesting that our brains respond differently to drinking in order to satiate thirst (a pleasant sensation) versus drinking after thirst has been satiated (an unpleasant experience). Furthermore, unlike camels, sheep, dogs and cows, who are able to quickly and accurately replace body-water deficits within five or ten minutes, we humans (along with guinea pigs, hamsters and rats) appear to be less efficient, with humans able to replace 50–80% of the deficit quite quickly, but repletion for the remainder occurring more slowly.

WHAT HAPPENS
WHEN YOU'RE DEHYDRATED?

Recognizing thirst is particularly crucial for people engaging in sport, a corner of the drinks market that is big business, with expensive hydrating drinks promising all kinds of secondary benefits. But what sounds like a simple process – recognizing and responding appropriately to thirst – can be difficult for more vulnerable sectors of the population: babies and infants, the elderly, or people with reduced kidney function.

Thirst arises as a result of dehydration, which in its most simple definition means "the process of losing water". When we're dehydrated, more water is moving out of our cells, or being lost to the body through sweating, than we are taking in. With water being so vital for our organs, the body reacts to dehydration by trying to conserve as much water as it can. The kidneys remove less water from the

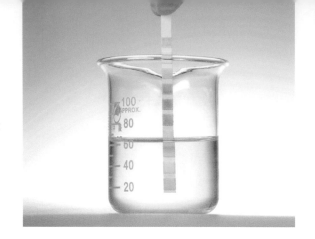

ABOVE: Pale, straw-coloured urine is a sign of good hydration.

blood and we urinate less often – and when we do the urine is darker in colour. Once a decreased level of dehydration is detected by the body, signals are sent to the brain to initiate the sensation of thirst.

Dehydration can arise as a result of physical

DOES CAFFEINE DEHYDRATE YOU?

A common perception is that caffeinated drinks dehydrate. This popular urban myth is so widely accepted that in 2016 the UK's Department of Health produced a leaflet for GP surgeries advising people on how to look after themselves in warm weather. They actually included the advice that people should avoid drinking caffeinated beverages in the heat! However, far from tea and coffee being dehydrating, the opposite is in fact true. Caffeine is found in tea, coffee, colas and some energy drinks at levels ranging from up to 40mg for some colas to 140mg for a mug of filter coffee. Overall, the evidence suggests that, while caffeine has a mild diuretic effect, consumption of up to about five mugs of filter coffee a day (500mg/day) does not

dehydrate. Rather, consumption of sugar-free tea or coffee can act as a low-calorie option for hydration. Pregnant ladies just need to be mindful to reduce intake to around 200mg/day, in line with medical recommendations, to avoid any risks relating to birth weight and growth.

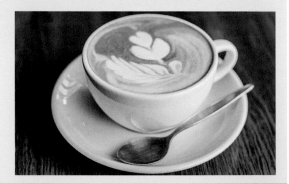

Nine signs of dehydration

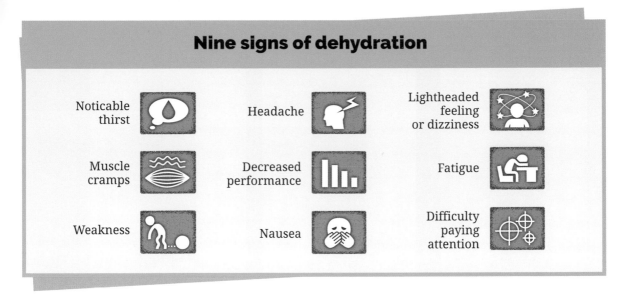

Noticable thirst

Headache

Lightheaded feeling or dizziness

Muscle cramps

Decreased performance

Fatigue

Weakness

Nausea

Difficulty paying attention

activity and exertion, whether recreational or through work, and can be exaggerated in hot or humid environments. It can also occur more easily at high altitudes and following prolonged periods of immersion, such as long-distance swimming in the sea. Dehydration of as little as 1–2% of body weight has been associated with adverse effects on mood, cognition, and mental and physical performance. Cue the role of thirst as our inbuilt sensor to tell us when the body detects that fluid is required.

Often the trigger for recognizing thirst is a dry mouth and throat, but this symptom typically only occurs after the kidneys have already begun to conserve water and concentrate urine, at around 1–2% loss of body weight, i.e. the level at which

the above adverse effects on function have been identified. Hence the debate as to whether thirst is an accurate indicator of hydration status and whether we should simply adhere to the daily intake guidance rather than relying on our own senses.

If you feel thirsty, then your body is certainly telling you to drink more. If you are in a hot environment, or are very hot from illness or from exercise, then you probably need to drink more in any case. A crude indicator of low hydration is dark-coloured urine during the day. Sports drinks are of most benefit following vigorous exercise for 45 minutes or thereabouts, and homemade versions work just as well as commercial ones for restoring hydration.

The bottom line: Being aware of your fluid needs and possibly even setting yourself a loose target of consuming around 1.5–2 litres (3 to 4 pints) of water or fluids each day is a good idea. You are likely to remain hydrated throughout the day and reap the associated benefits to health and performance. However, there is no need to get fixated on achieving a definitive amount because you think it will confer some kind of extra benefit. It's also worth remembering that many studies on dehydration and thirst have been conducted in environments where fluid and food intake was controlled: in real life, such circumstances are less likely. Most people can't even feel if they are mildly dehydrated and can cope with daily activities just as adequately as if they were properly hydrated. This is because our bodies are designed to maintain body-water balance, either by increasing or decreasing the sensation of thirst or by regulating urine output.

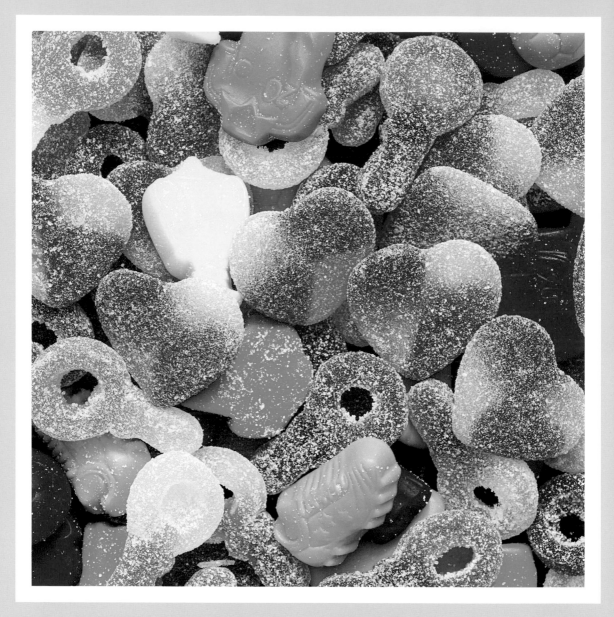

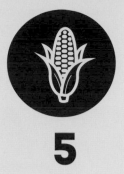

5

SWEET ENOUGH

Myths relating to foods containing carbohydrate and sugar, plus GI

CARBOHYDRATES: AN OVERVIEW

Although the "low-carb" diet has been fashionable since the 1970s, the amount of sugar we consume and the consequences of excess intake have only been hot topics in nutrition for the past few years.

Free sugars

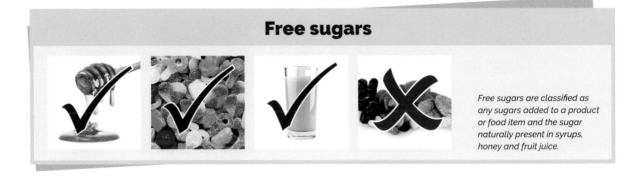

Free sugars are classified as any sugars added to a product or food item and the sugar naturally present in syrups, honey and fruit juice.

THE WORLD HEALTH ORGANIZATION published new guidelines on sugar intake in 2015, which urged governments to commit to reducing the intake of "free sugars" in adults and children. "Free sugars" include any sugar that's added to a product by manufacturers, cooks or consumers, or the sugar naturally present in syrups, honey and fruit juice. It doesn't include sugars in dairy products, nor in fresh or dried fruit as the sugar is held within the cell structure of the food.

In the US, the 2015–2020 Dietary Guidelines for Americans recommend restricting added sugars to no more than 10% of daily calories. Sugar consumption likewise rose up the UK public-health agenda in 2015, when the Scientific Advisory Committee on Nutrition (SACN) published its report "Carbohydrates and Health", which concluded that there is sufficient evidence of a direct link between sugar intake and obesity risk. In the report, SACN advised the government to reconsider its recommended daily intake of free sugars and to halve it to no more than 5% of daily energy intake. In more everyday terms, SACN said that adults (and children over 11) should be consuming no more than 30g (1oz, seven cubes) of sugar each day, children from 7 to 10 years should consume no more than 24g (0.9oz, six cubes) and children aged 4 to 6 years no more than 19g of free sugars (0.7oz, five cubes).

So how much are sugars, and more widely carbohydrates, responsible for our obesity epidemic? Are all carbohydrates bad for health or are there some types that we should be eating more of?

SHOULD YOU CUT ALL CARBS?

Carbohydrates include starches and sugars, as well as the fibre found in fruit, vegetables, pulses and grains. As one of the three macronutrients (the others being protein and fat), they are one of the three main ways in which the body obtains energy or calories.

IN FACT, CARBOHYDRATE IS the body's main source of energy for physical activity and is also needed by the brain. Starchy foods, particularly wholegrain foods, are also good sources of a number of important vitamins and minerals, as well as fibre.

In the UK, SACN extensively reviewed the evidence linking consumption of carbohydrate with health outcomes (looking at more than 600 peer-reviewed research papers). Although a high

sugar intake was linked with increased risk of dental caries and weight gain, a high fibre intake was crucially found to be beneficial for gut health and to help reduce the risk of heart disease, strokes, type 2 diabetes and colorectal cancer. Based on this evidence, the UK has new fibre recommendations: at least 30g (1oz) per day for adults; and for children, ages 2–5, 15g (0.5oz)/day; ages 5–11, 20g (0.7oz)/day; ages 11–16, 25g (0.9oz)/day; and ages 16–18, 30g/day.

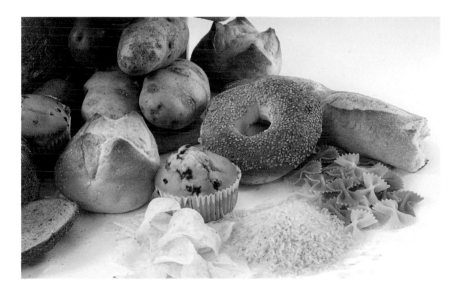

LEFT: These foods are avoided by those following low-carbohydrate diets.

DOES SUGAR MAKE YOU FAT?

There is good evidence that eating too much sugar can lead to weight gain. Humans have an innate desire for sweetness from birth, and sugar-containing foods, snacks and drinks are highly palatable and easy to consume in excess. However, it is important to remember that the underlying cause of obesity is energy imbalance – in other words, any source of excess calories can result in weight gain. Surveys reveal that our sugar consumption has been falling since around 2000, whilst obesity rates have continued to increase, suggesting that focusing on sugar alone isn't going to stop the epidemic.

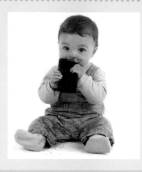

Meanwhile the European Food Safety Authority (EFSA) recommends 25g fibre per day for adults. Although fibre is often overlooked in much of the media coverage about carbohydrates, it is just as challenging to achieve, in the context of the dietary changes that most of us will need to make, as the new sugar recommendation.

So carbohydrates are still an important part of our diet – overall around 50% of our energy should come from carbohydrates. This means basing most of our meals on starchy foods. However, just as we have recognized that we need to think about the type as well as the amount of fat in our diets, the same is true for carbohydrates.

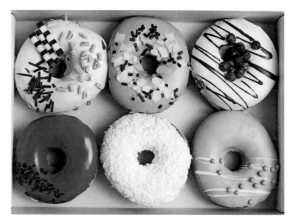

ABOVE: It is easier to overeat on doughnuts than on steaks.

The bottom line: There is widespread agreement that, on average, we eat too much sugar, and world health advice emphasizes that intake should be reduced. Foods high in free sugars can be high in energy and are often considered more palatable, therefore increasing the risk of excessive consumption, which in turn can lead to weight gain and obesity. But sugars are also naturally present in fruit, vegetables, milk and grains, and these are all foods that are important nutrient providers. So we should try to cut down on added sugars, for example in biscuits, cakes, confectionary, sugary drinks and breakfast cereals, but still eat plenty of fruit and vegetables and some lower-fat dairy products (preferably those without added sugars).

We should also replace refined carbs like white rice, pasta and bread with wholegrain and high-fibre foods. In practice, this means opting for brown rice and pasta, wholegrain breads and breakfast cereals, and potatoes in skins. We also need to eat plenty of other fibre-containing foods such as nuts, seeds and pulses.

CUT CARBS TO LOSE WEIGHT?

Low-carb diets have been popular in the Western world for some time; by nature they focus on reducing the amount of carbohydrate in the diet to promote weight loss.

MANY PEOPLE THINK OF the low-carb diet as a "fad" diet, but it shows little sign of falling out of favour, having become popular as the Atkins diet in the early 1970s. Recent forms of the low-carb diet include the "new" Atkins diet, the Zone diet and the Palaeo diet, which are fairly similar in their basis.

Low-carb diets usually restrict carbohydrates to less than 20% of energy intake. These diets are not just low in carbs – they are also high in protein and often also fat. Studies have shown that this approach can help some people to lose weight in the short term, and this is probably because protein helps to keep you feeling full, which can help appetite control. For example, a study published in the New England Journal of Medicine found that people who ate a low-carb diet lost more weight than those receiving a conventional "low-fat" diet for the first six months. There have now been a number of trials, mostly in people with health problems, including those who are obese or have type 2 diabetes, and the majority have shown the low-carb diet to do better than a low-fat diet at the beginning.

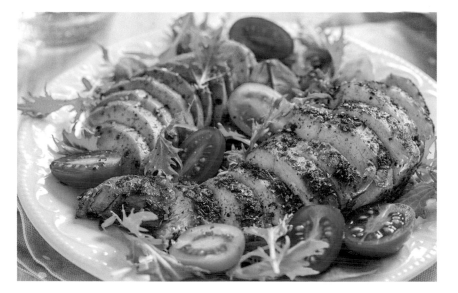

LEFT: Protein can help to increase a feeling of fullness (satiety) and remove the desire to continue eating (satiation).

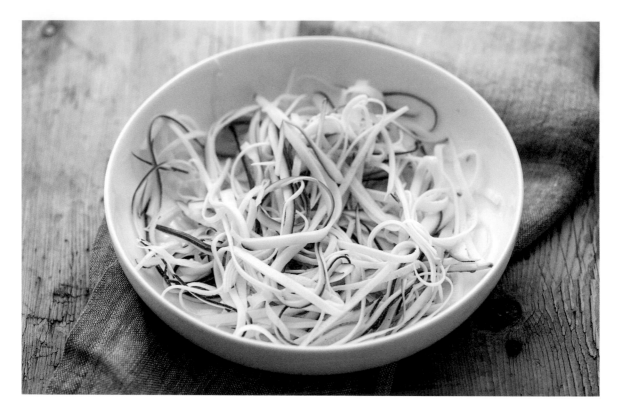

Although longer-term studies are more limited, those that have compared weight loss on calorie-controlled low-carb and low-fat diets over at least a year have generally found little difference between them. In other words, different weight-loss strategies are effective in different people, particularly over a prolonged period.

Concerns also remain about the safety of this type of dietary pattern in the long term. Cutting out a whole food group may result in a diet that does not contain all the nutrients the body needs, for instance, especially since cutting carbs inevitably leads to a low fibre intake, which can have an adverse effect on gut health. Eating high-fat foods may lead to a high intake of saturated fat, which is linked to increased risk of heart disease. The high animal-protein content of many of these types of diets is also at odds with current advice to consume more sustainable, plant-based sources of protein,

like beans, lentils, pulses, nuts and Quorn. So most experts agree that low-carb diets should, if anything, be considered as a temporary weight-loss tool rather than a "diet for life".

Carbohydrate is an important source of energy for the body – which is why low-carb diets can lead to headaches and fatigue – but starchy foods are not fattening per se. Weight gain typically results from eating more calories than your body uses, and these calories can be from any source – protein, fat, carbohydrate or alcohol. (Carbohydrate contains 4kcal/g compared to fat, which contains 9kcal/g; 1g = 0.035oz.) However, starchy foods are sometimes combined with high-fat ingredients, e.g. butter on bread or creamy sauces with pasta, and this makes them much higher in calories. But provided starchy foods are not cooked or served with a lot of fat, and portion sizes are moderate, they are relatively low in calories.

Low-carb diets and type 2 diabetes

SACN concluded that the proportion of carbohydrate in the diet has no effect on the risk of developing type 2 diabetes. But there has been a lot of interest in the role of low-carb in managing type 2 diabetes. The amount, type and frequency of carbohydrate-containing foods in a diet is very important for blood-glucose management, and including low-glycaemic-index (GI) carbohydrate foods within a healthy, balanced diet can be a strategy to help them with blood-sugar control (see page 73). And because 90% of people with type 2 diabetes are obese or overweight, low-carb diets can also aid weight loss. Nonetheless, the experts suggest that while low-carb diets can help some people, there is no consistent evidence that they have any advantage over other diets in the long term (Diabetes UK, 2016).

Many diets that include low-carbohydrate, Mediterranean, low-fat or very low-calorie foods can help people lose or manage their weight, and the choice should be based on individual food preferences and lifestyles – what's most important is being able to stick to the diet over a long period. Before making any dietary changes to reduce carbohydrate intake, people with type 2 diabetes should always seek medical advice, as dietary changes may require alterations to medication.

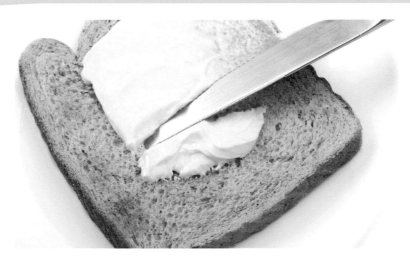

OPPOSITE ABOVE: Shredded veg such as courgetti and cauli rice have become fashionable replacements for pasta and rice.

RIGHT: Bread is a good source of carbohydrate, but a thick spreading of butter makes this meal high in fat.

The bottom line: The main reason why a low-carb diet may be effective for weight loss seems to be related to the relatively high protein content of these diets rather than the lack of carbohydrate. So rather than focusing on cutting out carbohydrates if you are trying to lose weight, it is a better idea to include lean, protein-rich foods like lean meats, skinless chicken, fish, low-fat dairy products and pulses in your main meals. Including wholegrain carbohydrate foods will also provide more fibre, which can be helpful for weight loss too.

SHOULD YOU ONLY EAT LOW-GI FOODS?

The carbohydrates in food are present in various forms, such as molecules of starch or simple sugars. During digestion they are broken down into glucose (and other single sugars) so that they can be absorbed into the body.

Carbohydrate molecules

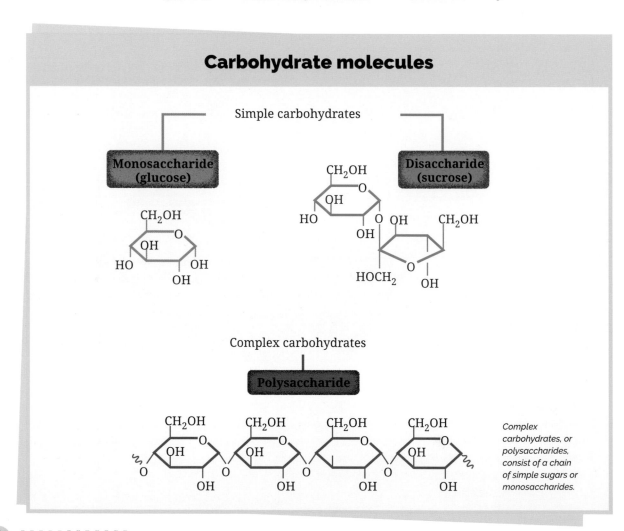

Simple carbohydrates

Monosaccharide (glucose)

Disaccharide (sucrose)

Complex carbohydrates

Polysaccharide

Complex carbohydrates, or polysaccharides, consist of a chain of simple sugars or monosaccharides.

THE GLYCAEMIC INDEX (GI) of a food is a measure of how quickly the glucose gets absorbed into the bloodstream after eating. The more quickly glucose is absorbed, the higher the level of glucose in the blood, and this gives the food a higher GI score.

Of course, most foods do not just exist as pure carbohydrate; other components are present too, including fat, protein and fibre, and these will have an effect on the GI score, as will the processing of the food and the cooking method. Indeed, these factors can have such an impact that it is not safe to make assumptions based on the GIs of various foods. For example, both apples and apple juice have a low GI, whereas orange juice has a higher GI.

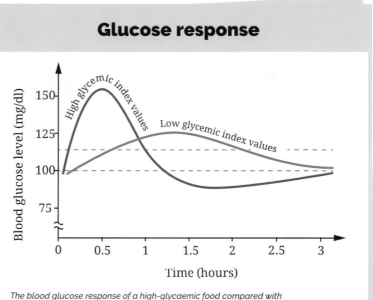

Glucose response

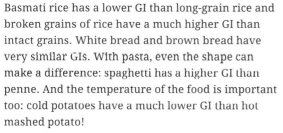

The blood glucose response of a high-glycaemic food compared with a low-glycaemic food.

Basmati rice has a lower GI than long-grain rice and broken grains of rice have a much higher GI than intact grains. White bread and brown bread have very similar GIs. With pasta, even the shape can make a difference: spaghetti has a higher GI than penne. And the temperature of the food is important too: cold potatoes have a much lower GI than hot mashed potato!

Despite some of these quirks, foods with a low GI generally tend to contain a greater amount of fibre and be less processed, so it is thought that choosing lower-GI foods is better for health; there are plenty of books and diet plans based on this principle. Low-GI diets are sometimes recommended for people with diabetes, as they can help them to keep their blood-glucose levels more stable, but the regime must be followed in the context of an overall balanced diet and not based solely on the GI score of each individual food. As we have seen, using the glycaemic index can be misleading as GI alone does not determine whether a food is a healthy choice. High-fat foods like chocolate and pastries have a lower GI than rice or pasta, but this doesn't make them healthier!

The bottom line: A diet that consists mainly of low-GI foods can keep blood-sugar levels stable and therefore help to manage appetite and weight, and may also help to reduce the risk of type 2 diabetes and heart disease. But rather than obsessing over the GI of each food, it is better to choose wholegrains over refined grains (quinoa rather than white rice, for instance) and to eat starchy foods with more fibre (Weetabix rather than Corn Flakes).

DO FIZZY DRINKS CAUSE OBESITY?

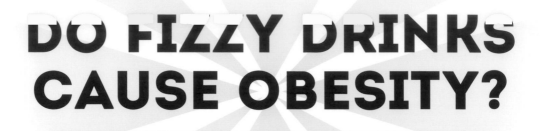

Drinks make a significant contribution to calorie and sugar intakes for many people, particularly children and adolescents. Non-alcoholic drinks (including soft drinks and fruit juices) provide around a quarter of our daily intake of free sugars (the type we are advised to cut back on). A can (330ml/11fl oz) of cola alone provides 35g (1.2oz) of sugar and 139 calories.

....

BELOW: While fizzy drinks don't provide any health benefits, they cannot be held solely accountable for causing obesity.

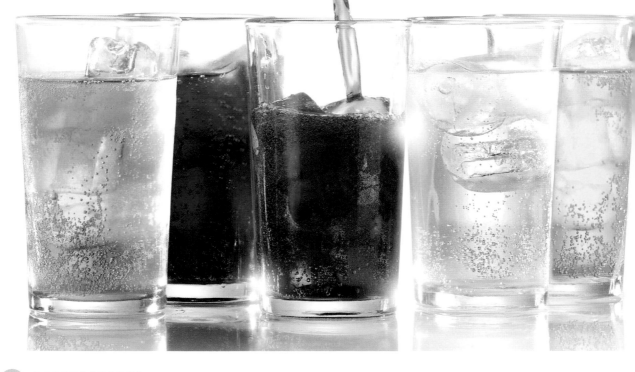

The sugar content of soft drinks

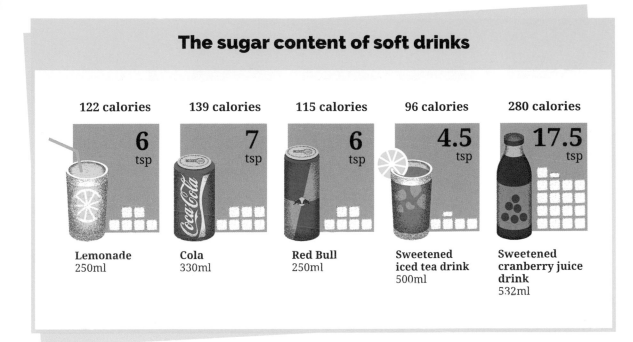

122 calories	139 calories	115 calories	96 calories	280 calories
6 tsp	**7** tsp	**6** tsp	**4.5** tsp	**17.5** tsp
Lemonade 250ml	Cola 330ml	Red Bull 250ml	Sweetened iced tea drink 500ml	Sweetened cranberry juice drink 532ml

THE SCIENTIFIC COMMUNITY IS somewhat split when it comes to the debate over calories from liquids, and it has been suggested by some that liquid calories aren't as filling as calories from solid food. So, for example, if you drink a can of fizzy drink that supplies approximately 140 calories, you would not feel the need to offset those calories by eating less at a later meal, but had you eaten two biscuits, you might be more likely to compensate for the calories by eating less later. This may be too simplistic because other factors are often involved, but certainly it is easy to consume a significant number of calories very quickly by drinking sugary beverages. While fruit juice contains vitamins and minerals, soft drinks offer little or no nutritional benefit. As well as increasing risk of tooth decay by sugar, frequent consumption of fizzy drinks can lead to dental erosion due to the acids present, which is why these types of drinks are not advised for children. Concern about their contribution to energy intakes has led some European countries, Mexico and several US states to announce a tax on them.

Current advice from bodies such as the Department of Health in the UK and the United States Department of Agriculture is to swap sugary fizzy drinks for water (including sparkling water), lower-fat milks or sugar-free, diet and no-added-sugar drinks. Nevertheless, headlines continue to suggest that diet drinks themselves may not offer any benefit for weight loss – or may even be linked to weight gain. So have the experts now changed their minds?

If you look at the advice of leading organizations like Diabetes UK, the American Heart Association and the British Dietetic Association, the answer to this is "no". Studies that look at what people consume and follow them over time have shown mixed results, some of them indeed linking low-calorie drinks with obesity. The problem with relying on findings from this type of study is that the relationship may have been affected by overweight people being more likely to choose low-calorie options. Studies that have compared the effects of sugary drinks and low-calorie drinks on calorie intake and weight over time have found that the low-calorie drinks lead to a lower calorie intake and eventual weight loss.

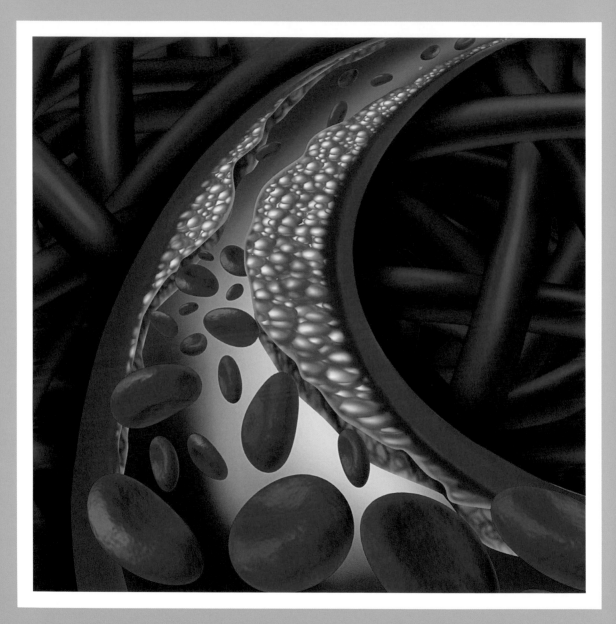

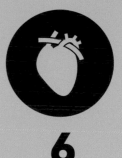

6

EAT FAT, GET FAT

Myths relating to the consumption
of fats and high-cholesterol foods

TYPES OF FAT IN THE DIET: AN OVERVIEW

The nature of a fat depends on the types of fatty acids it is made up of. All dietary sources of fat contain both saturated and unsaturated fatty acids, but they are often described as either "saturated fat" or "unsaturated fat" according to the proportions of fatty acids present.

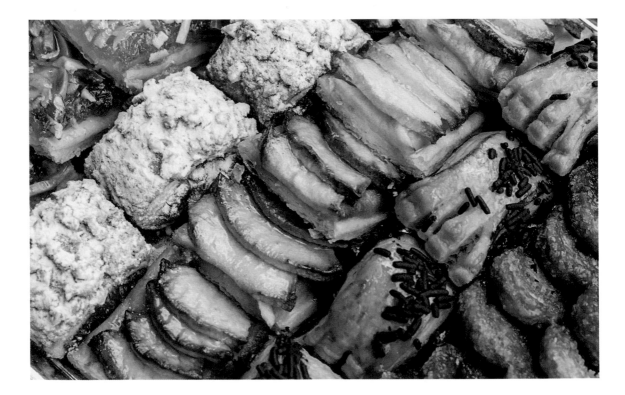

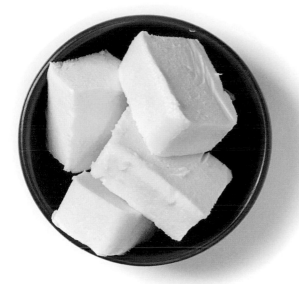

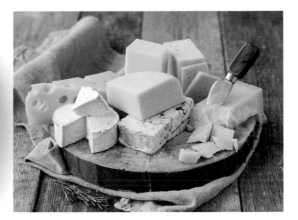

FOR EXAMPLE, BUTTER IS often described as a saturated fat because it has more saturated fatty acids than it does unsaturated fatty acids, while most vegetable oils are described as unsaturated fats as they contain a higher proportion of these. It is now well recognized that the balance of fatty acids, rather than the amount of fat in the diet, is the most important consideration in terms of health.

TYPES OF FAT

Saturated fat comes mainly from animal sources of food, such as butter, fatty red meats and processed meats, and full-fat dairy products. Saturated fat raises blood cholesterol levels (the "bad" form of blood cholesterol known as LDL-cholesterol) and high intakes have been linked with increased risk of heart disease, stroke and type 2 diabetes.

Trans fat occurs naturally in some foods, in very small amounts, but most trans fats are made from oils through a food-processing method called partial hydrogenation, which is used to "harden" vegetable oils to form a semi-solid. Partially hydrogenated trans fats can be used in food manufacturing to improve shelf life and the culinary properties of foods, and were once common constituents of margarines and spreads. However, they have been shown to increase

OPPOSITE: Pastries made with butter or other animal fats have a high saturated-fat content.

ABOVE LEFT & ABOVE: Butter and cheese are among the prime sources of saturated fat.

LDL-cholesterol even more than saturated fats and concern about their health effects has led to changes in manufacturing practices in recent years. As a result, good progress has been made in removing these fatty acids from our food; for example, fat spreads sold in the UK no longer contain partially hydrogenated vegetable oil. This has led to the average trans-fatty-acid content of the UK diet falling well below the recommended upper limit and many foods are now entirely free of trans fats.

The potentially "healthy" dietary fats are the unsaturated ones. These include monounsaturated and polyunsaturated fats, both of which have been shown to reduce blood cholesterol levels when they replace saturated fat in the diet.

Monounsaturated fats are found in high amounts in olive, peanut and rapeseed oils, avocados, nuts and seeds such as pumpkin and sesame seeds.

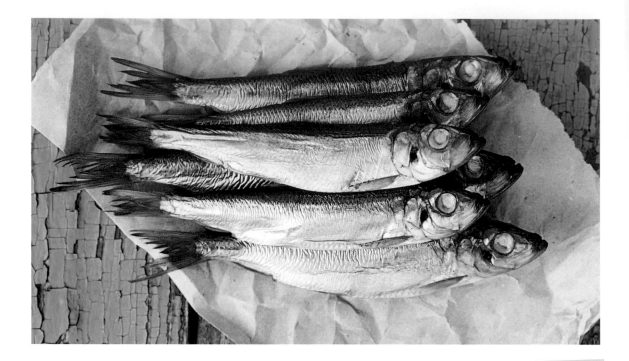

Polyunsaturated fats are found mostly in plant-based foods and oils such as sunflower oil, sesame oil, soya oil and spreads made from these, as well as in flaxseeds, pine nuts, sesame seeds, sunflower seeds and walnuts. Omega-3 fatty acids are a type of polyunsaturated fatty acid that have been shown to reduce the risk of heart disease. The best source of these fatty acids is oily fish (e.g. sardines, salmon and mackerel), which is why dietary guidelines recommend regular consumption of oily fish.

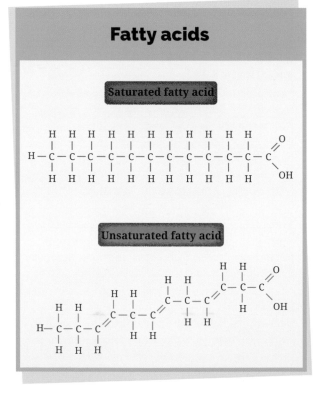

ABOVE & RIGHT: Oily fish is a good source of polyunsaturated fats while avocados contain mainly monounsaturated fat.

Fatty acids

Saturated fatty acid

Unsaturated fatty acid

DOES EATING FAT MAKE YOU FAT?

There has been a great deal of controversy in recent years about whether the long-standing advice that people reduce their intake of fat, particularly saturated fat, in order to lower their risk of heart disease, has been misplaced.

THIS ADVICE, FROM BOTH national and international bodies including the World Health Organization, developed from two sources: animal studies showing that diets high in saturated fat led to fatty deposits accumulating in the arteries; and population studies, such as the famous Seven Countries Study, which was set up to monitor the correlation between diet, lifestyle and health, showing that populations with high saturated-fat intakes had the highest rates of heart disease. It is now widely accepted from laboratory studies that a high intake of saturated fat leads to raised levels of blood cholesterol, high levels of which are a risk factor for heart disease. As fat is the most concentrated form of dietary energy (providing 9kcal/g compared to 3.75kcal/g for carbohydrates and 4kcal/g for protein, see page 44), foods that contain a lot of fat provide a lot of calories. Low-fat diets are therefore promoted as much for weight loss as for cholesterol control.

Since the 1970s, the food industry has responded to public concern about fat by developing a wide range of "low-fat" and "fat-free" products, including lower-fat milks and other dairy products, low-fat spreads and lower-fat ready meals. Sales of these products have rocketed.

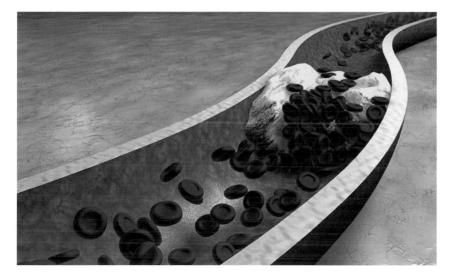

LEFT: Cross section of an artery clogged with a cholesterol plaque blocking the flow of blood.

DOES FAT REALLY DESERVE ITS BAD REPUTATION?

Virtually all natural foods contain some fat because both plants and animals use fat as the most economical way to store energy. It is needed for growth, proper functioning of the nerves and brain, maintaining healthy skin and other tissues, transporting the fat-soluble vitamins (A, D, E and K) through the bloodstream to where they are required, and forming the hormones needed to regulate many bodily processes. Some essential functions are performed by dietary fats that we can't produce in our bodies (we cannot form the omega-3 fatty acid alpha-linolenic acid or the omega-6 fatty acid linoleic acid), so we actually need some fat from our diet to survive. So, as with most things, too much fat can be detrimental, but a certain amount is compatible with good health.

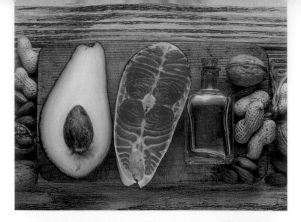

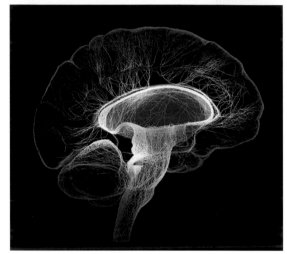

ABOVE RIGHT: Good sources of healthy fats include avocados, oily fish and nuts.

RIGHT: The brain and its network of nerves rely on fat as a vital component in order to function healthily.

The bottom line: Low-fat diets have been promoted for weight loss for many years, although comparisons with other diets suggest that it is energy intake that determines the extent of weight loss, rather than the relative proportions of macronutrients (fat, protein or carbohydrate) in the diet. Portion-size control is therefore an important part of any weight-loss strategy.

The success or failure of any diet depends on how well people adhere to it – and this in turn depends on more than just the macronutrient composition of the diet (e.g. the amount of fat): also important are issues of palatability, convenience and satiety (feeling of fullness). Different individuals will therefore find success through different approaches, especially in the long term.

The increase in low-fat foods on the market in recent years has improved access to such foods, helping many more people to follow low-fat diets. Others, however, find such products less palatable and do better adhering to a moderate-fat diet, which can still be high in fibre-rich foods such as wholegrains, fruit and vegetables. In addition, some fat-containing foods, such as nuts, have been shown to help with appetite control by influencing satiety; this is very important in long-term weight loss as many dieters blame their lack of success on feelings of hunger when following certain regimes.

DO SATURATED FATS CAUSE HEART DISEASE?

There is convincing evidence from many trials that saturated fatty acids can raise blood cholesterol levels, while replacing them with unsaturated fatty acids or wholegrains can reduce "bad" LDL-cholesterol. There is also strong evidence linking high LDL-cholesterol levels with an increased risk of heart disease – we know, for example, that use of statin drugs to lower LDL-cholesterol reduces risk of a heart attack. However, some studies that have measured fat intake and followed participants over time have not been able to show a relationship between their saturated-fat intake and their risk of suffering a heart attack. This is perhaps not surprising as one measurement of someone's diet is not a good assessment of their fat intake over a long period, particularly as the fat content of our food supply has changed so much in recent years.

That said, the relationship between saturated fatty acids and heart health does seem to be more complex than the widely accepted message that "saturated fatty acids are bad". For one thing, there are different types of saturated fatty acids that seem to have different effects on blood cholesterol, so the types of foods eaten will affect whether there is an increased risk. Moreover, and very importantly, it depends on what replaces the saturated fatty acids in a person's diet – replacing saturated fats with refined carbohydrates doesn't seem to offer any benefit, while replacing them with unsaturated fats or complex carbohydrates (e.g. from wholegrain foods) does. This has not been

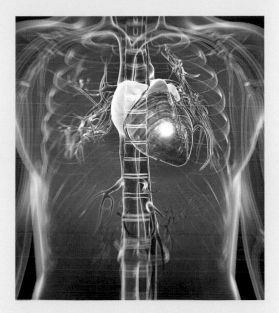

ABOVE: *Heart disease, with attendant blocked arteries, is the leading cause of heart attacks..*

reflected in much of the recent press coverage relating to this issue.

The most convincing evidence comes from a systematic review of randomized controlled trials involving almost 60,000 people, which concluded that reducing dietary saturated fatty acids can lower the risk of cardiovascular events by 17% (Hooper *et al.*, 2015). The authors suggested that lifestyle advice should continue to include a reduction in intake of saturated fatty acids, and partial replacement of these with unsaturated fatty acids.

IS OLIVE OIL ALWAYS THE HEALTHIEST CHOICE?

Olive oil is a key feature of the Mediterranean diet, a diet which is associated with good heart health and a lower risk of heart disease. All oils are a mixture of saturated and unsaturated fatty acids, but olive oil is relatively high in unsaturated – particularly monounsaturated – fatty acids (see graph).

THE REALITY IS that, as well as containing olive oil, a Mediterranean diet consists of fruits and vegetables, seafood, grains and other foods that are often credited with fighting against heart disease as well as some cancers and type 2 diabetes, so it is very difficult to deduce the individual contribution of each.

Most dietary advice involves swapping foods high in saturated fats for those rich in unsaturated fats. In the UK, the government's Eatwell Guide advocates consuming small amounts of unsaturated oils (plant and vegetables oils such as rapeseed, olive and nut oils, and spreads made from them) and using those with a high proportion of saturated fats sparingly. These latter include coconut oil, goose fat, ghee and butter, which can be used for flavour but in limited amounts. Palm oil is also high in saturated fat.

Scientists have discovered that heating up vegetable oils releases high concentrations of chemicals called aldehydes, and there is some concern that these, in high doses, could potentially be linked with cancer. These harmful aldehydes are released when an oil starts to smoke. Therefore oils with high smoke points (e.g. sunflower, standard rapeseed or olive and peanut oils) are better for roasting and frying, whereas those with lower smoke points (e.g. virgin oils, walnut and hempseed oils) are better kept for salad dressing or drizzling. Refined oils, such as sunflower and soy, have a higher smoke point than virgin/cold-pressed oils, and so are more suitable for high-temperature cooking.

COCONUT OIL – THE BEST FAT BY FAR?

Coconut oil has been heralded by health blogs and the popular press as a cure-all product with a wide range of health benefits including weight reduction, lowered cholesterol and quicker wound healing, as well as having a positive effect on the immune system, energy and memory. Due to its perception as a health-enhancing ingredient, some food manufacturers have now started to include coconut oil in their products in order to use it as a unique selling point. However, coconut oil contains around 90% saturated fat, which is by far the highest proportion out of all the edible oils and fats, including palm oil (50%), butter (52%) and lard (40%). What's more, studies have shown coconut oil to raise blood cholesterol levels.

In its defence, coconut oil – particularly extra-virgin coconut oil – has been found to contain compounds known as polyphenols, which various studies have deemed to be good for health. But polyphenols are also found in fruits and vegetables, which obviously also contain vitamins, minerals and fibre, and are therefore healthier sources of these compounds.

Around 65% of the fatty acids in coconut oil are known as "medium-chain" fatty acids due to their chemical structure. These fatty acids are thought to be metabolized slightly differently from other types of fatty acids in our bodies, and this is why coconut-oil advocates claim eating it can help you lose weight. However, human studies testing medium-chain fatty acids have had variable results in terms of the effect on body weight, and it is important to remember that coconut oil also contains other types of fatty acids. There are very few human studies that have measured the effect of coconut oil itself on weight loss, and those that have been published are of poor quality, so at the moment there is no good evidence

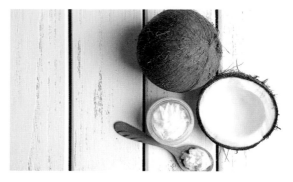

ABOVE: Despite its high saturated-fat content, the use of coconut oil is a growing trend.

to support this claim. Additionally, there is no evidence that coconut oil keeps you full for longer than other fats or that it speeds up metabolic rate.

Coconut oil can be used sparingly to flavour foods but should be consumed in small quantities. Hydrogenated coconut oil should be avoided completely as some brands contain trans-fatty acids, which are known to be particularly harmful.

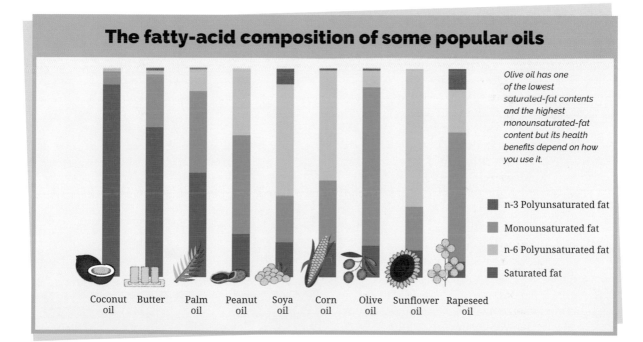

The fatty-acid composition of some popular oils

Olive oil has one of the lowest saturated-fat contents and the highest monounsaturated-fat content but its health benefits depend on how you use it.

- n-3 Polyunsaturated fat
- Monounsaturated fat
- n-6 Polyunsaturated fat
- Saturated fat

Coconut oil | Butter | Palm oil | Peanut oil | Soya oil | Corn oil | Olive oil | Sunflower oil | Rapeseed oil

A microscope image of fatty acids extracted from human fat.

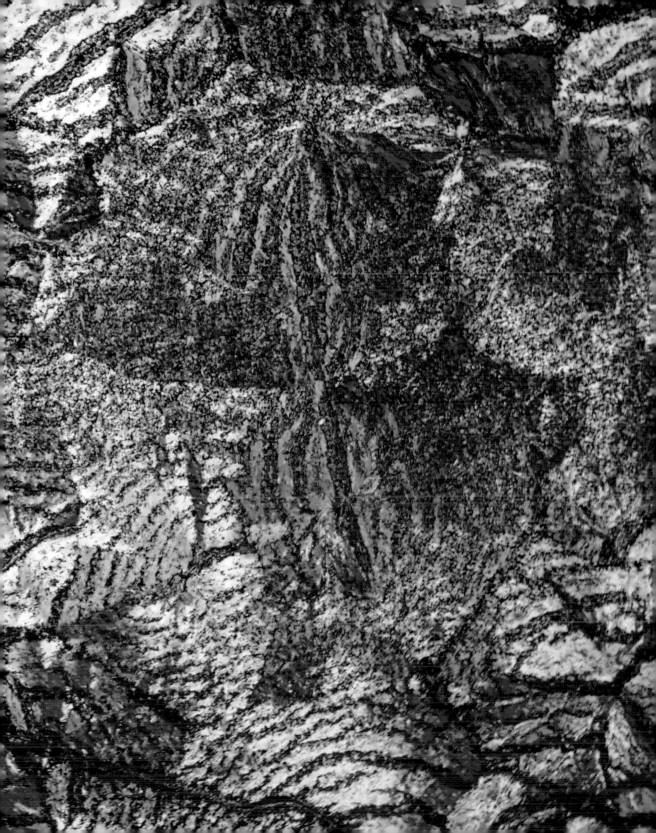

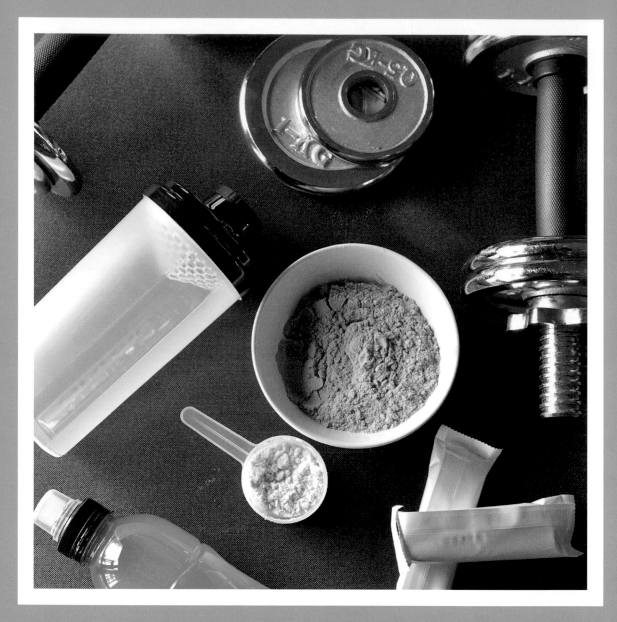

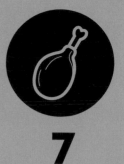

7

THE BUILDING BLOCKS OF LIFE

Myths relating to the consumption of protein

PROTEIN: AN OVERVIEW

Protein is needed for the growth, repair and renewal of cells. It has structural and functional roles within every cell in the body and is involved in a wide range of biological processes that keep us alive and healthy. After water, protein is the most abundant substance in the body. Nearly 50% of protein in the body is in the form of muscles, and there are substantial amounts in the skin and blood too. Protein also provides the body with energy.

PROTEINS ARE LARGE MOLECULES made up of long chains of amino acids, often referred to as building blocks. There are about 20 different amino acids commonly found in plant and animal proteins and the structure and function of these different types of protein depend on the sequence and characteristics of the constituent amino acids.

Amino acids are categorized as indispensable, conditionally indispensable and dispensable. Indispensable amino acids are essential in the diet as they cannot be made in the body, whereas

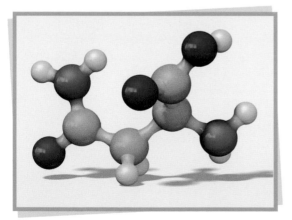

dispensable amino acids can be converted in the body from the indispensable ones.

Conditionally indispensable amino acids are needed in the diets of children because, while they are young, they are unable to make enough to meet their needs. Certain amino acids can become conditionally indispensable for adults during times of severe trauma or disease, or during periods of intense training.

A protein can also be categorized as high or low quality, depending on the types and quantities of amino acids it is made up of. Proteins from animal sources are considered to have a higher biological value than proteins from plant sources. This is because they tend to contain greater amounts of indispensable amino acids, since the patterns of amino acids in animal cells is comparable to the pattern in human cells. In comparison, plant foods tend to have very different patterns. However, vegans and strict vegetarians are still able to meet their requirement of indispensable amino acids by eating a combination of plant proteins that have a complementary effect, boosting their overall biological value. Good sources of plant protein

Types of amino acid

INDISPENSABLE AMINO ACIDS	CONDITIONALLY INDISPENSABLE AMINO ACIDS	DISPENSABLE AMINO ACIDS
LEUCINE	ARGININE	SERINE
ISOLEUCINE	HISTIDINE	ALANINE
VALINE	CYSTEINE	ASPARAGINE
THREONINE	GLYCINE	GLUTAMIC ACID
METHIONINE	TYROSINE	ASPARTIC ACID
PHENYLALANINE	GLUTAMINE	
TRYPTOPHAN	PROLINE	
LYSINE		

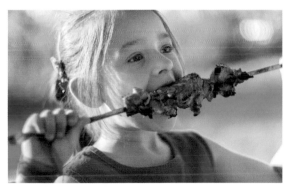

OPPOSITE: A model of a molecule of the amino acid asparagine, found in animal and plant protein sources.

ABOVE: Meat is considered a source of high-quality protein as it provides adequate amounts of all the essential amino acids.

RIGHT: Bread is not considered a high-quality-protein food as it may be lacking in one or more of the essential amino acids; but other foods, such as baked beans, can provide complementary amino acids,

include nuts, seeds, pulses, mycoprotein (fungal protein, found in Quorn) and soya products. There are also various amounts in grains such as quinoa.

The processing of foods may have an effect on some amino acids. When bread is toasted or foods are baked, for instance, the browning that occurs reduces the availability of the indispensable amino acid lysine.

The main sources of protein include meat, fish, eggs, milk, cheese, cereals, bread, nuts and pulses.

The current recommended dietary allowance is 0.8g (0.3oz) of protein per kilogram of body weight. This equates to approximately 56g (2oz) per day for men and 45g (1.6oz) per day for women, though relatively more is required by pregnant and breastfeeding women.

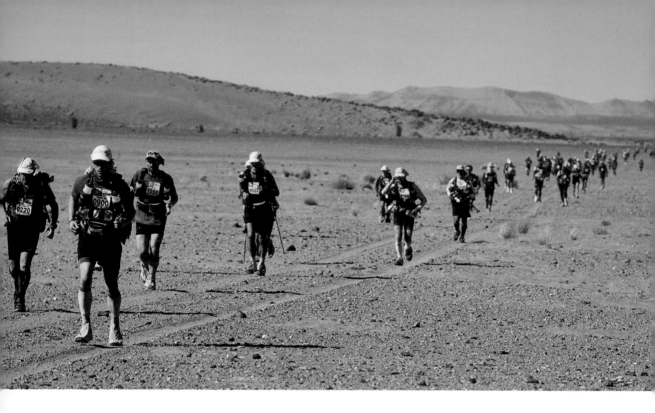

Protein intakes higher than this are often advocated by those involved in sport or the diet industry, despite the lack of evidence that greater amounts are needed.

One exception is ultra-endurance athletes, who need increased protein intakes for recovery from intense exercise such as Ironman triathlons. Studies suggest that the dietary protein intake necessary to support protein balance in the body of endurance athletes ranges from 1.2 to 1.4g (c.0.4–0.5oz) of protein per kilogram of body weight per day. Recent studies have shown that protein turnover may become more efficient in response to endurance exercise training, so this recommendation could drop to 1g (c.0.35oz) for those who compete on a regular basis. Ultra-endurance athletes who engage in continuous activity for many hours or consecutive days of intermittent exercise (such as the Marathon des Sables, a six-day ultramarathon in the Sahara Desert) should also consume protein at or slightly above 1.2–1.4g.

ABOVE: Participants in the Marathon de Sables, running ultra distances over six days, carry their own food, so careful planning is required to ensure sufficient calorific intake, in particular from protein.

Resistance exercise may necessitate a higher-than-average protein intake (i.e. in excess of 0.8g/0.3oz) because additional protein, and in particular certain essential amino acids known as branched-chain amino acids, are needed for the repair and growth of muscles after high-intensity exercise. These branched-chain amino acids are most useful in the early phases of strength training, when the most significant gains in muscle size occur. However, as in endurance exercise training, when an individual trains more and protein use becomes more efficient, the amount of protein needed to maintain muscle mass may drop. Recommended protein intakes for strength-trained athletes range from approximately 1.2 up to 1.7g per kilogram (0.5–0.8oz per lb) of body weight per day for the biggest bodybuilders.

The impact of resistance exercise on muscle protein

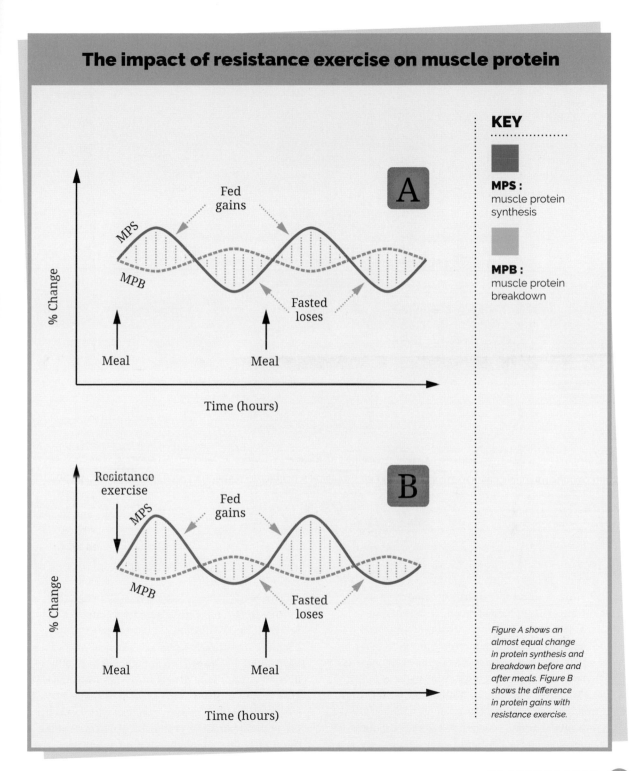

KEY

MPS : muscle protein synthesis

MPB : muscle protein breakdown

Figure A shows an almost equal change in protein synthesis and breakdown before and after meals. Figure B shows the difference in protein gains with resistance exercise.

Protein metabolism

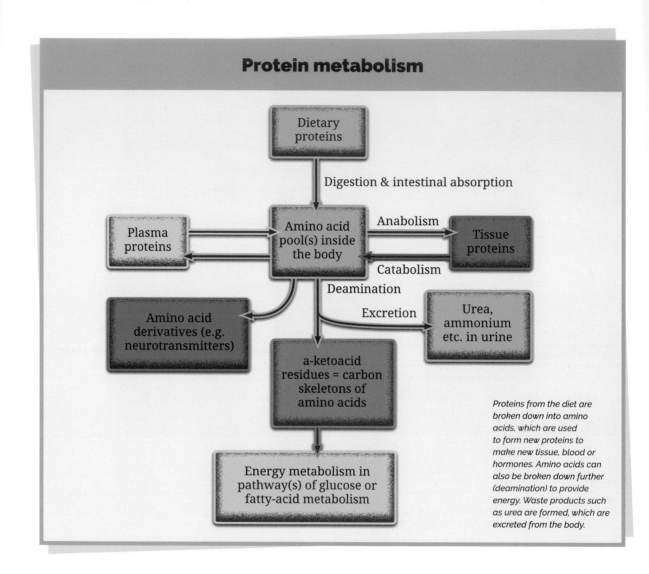

Dietary proteins

Digestion & intestinal absorption

Plasma proteins

Amino acid pool(s) inside the body

Anabolism

Tissue proteins

Catabolism

Deamination

Excretion

Amino acid derivatives (e.g. neurotransmitters)

Urea, ammonium etc. in urine

a-ketoacid residues = carbon skeletons of amino acids

Energy metabolism in pathway(s) of glucose or fatty-acid metabolism

Proteins from the diet are broken down into amino acids, which are used to form new proteins to make new tissue, blood or hormones. Amino acids can also be broken down further (deamination) to provide energy. Waste products such as urea are formed, which are excreted from the body.

Numerous studies have compared the relative effectiveness of individual amino acids for the maintenance, repair and building of muscle in response to training, but recent studies focusing on whole protein (as opposed to amino acids) such as whey, casein and soya have found these to be just as effective. The timing of the consumption of these proteins or amino acids is an important factor in their effectiveness, and research shows they should be consumed just before or just after strength exercise to achieve net gains in muscle. As well as timing, another important consideration is the amount of protein taken. While it might be tempting to knock back a couple of shakes and a chicken leg, studies have found that there is an optimum dose of 20–25g (0.7–0.9oz) of protein to maximally stimulate muscle growth after exercise. A lower amount results in suboptimal rates of protein synthesis whereas much bigger doses stimulate protein breakdown, negating the effects of the simultaneous protein synthesis.

DO HIGH-PROTEIN DIETS MAKE YOU LOSE WEIGHT?

Protein-rich foods tend to make people feel fuller than foods rich in carbohydrates or fat. So including a lean source of protein in a meal can help minimize feelings of hunger and decrease overall energy intake.

HOWEVER, SOME SELF-STYLED "diet coaches" advocate up to 200g (7oz) of protein per day from a combination of powders and animal-protein foods. This is nearly four times the amount actually needed by the body.

Some studies have shown protein-rich diets with a low carbohydrate content to be associated with a greater initial weight loss compared with other types of diets, such as low-fat. However, this effect is lost over time and few or no differences have generally been reported when comparisons have been made after a couple of months.

Experiencing substantial weight loss at the beginning of a diet can be very motivational at first, but high-protein diets are difficult to stick to as they are often too restrictive, repetitive and impractical for most people's lifestyles. They tend to feature a great deal of chicken and turkey!

Weight loss will only occur if a negative energy balance is achieved: that is, a deficit in energy intake compared to output through activity. Large amounts of protein add more calories (energy) to the diet. A higher proportion of protein within the context of a lower-calorie intake may achieve the best weight-loss results, but that is not the same as eating unlimited amounts of protein.

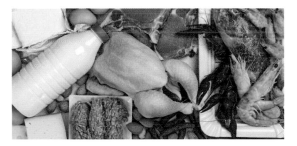

ABOVE: High-protein foods include eggs, milk, chicken, pork, fish and seafood.

The bottom line: High-protein diets tend to produce great weight loss results to begin with, but their restrictive nature makes them difficult to stick to long-term. It has to be remembered that weight loss results from achieving a deficit in energy intake and energy expenditure, so a couch potato gorging on steaks and sausages in unlikely to see any results!

SHOULD YOU DRINK PROTEIN SHAKES FOR BIG MUSCLES?

A client recently came to me with a large bucket of protein powder and was keen for me to reassure him he hadn't wasted his money. The answer is not a clear yes or no. No longer confined to the realm of extreme bodybuilding, protein shakes are now hugely popular in all types of sport and exercise.

THERE ARE A NUMBER of different types of protein shakes available and while the majority contain whey protein in various forms, other brands use soya, hemp, rice and pea protein to make them suitable for vegetarians and vegans.

Most people wrongly assume that protein shakes act as a bulking agent to build big muscles, whereas what they really do is deliver important amino acids to muscles to help them repair and recover after a strenuous workout. Protein shakes also contain carbohydrate to help replenish depleted energy stores within the muscle. While they can be useful when used at the right time, excessive use or use on days when no exercise has been performed just results in extra calorie intake, which, if not offset by activity, will result in fat gain.

Whey is the most common base for the protein powder, as it contains a higher proportion of the branched-chain amino acids that have been found to facilitate the healing of damaged muscles.

The whey protein added to shakes comes in three different forms: isolates, hydrolysates and

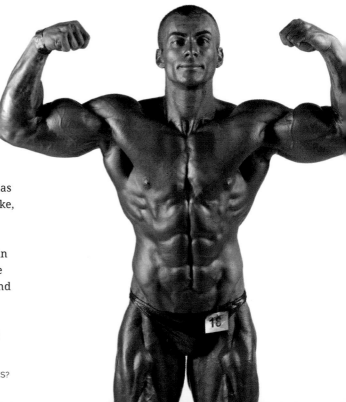

BELOW: Muscle mass can be built through a combination of resistance training and a diet providing adequate amounts of amino acids.

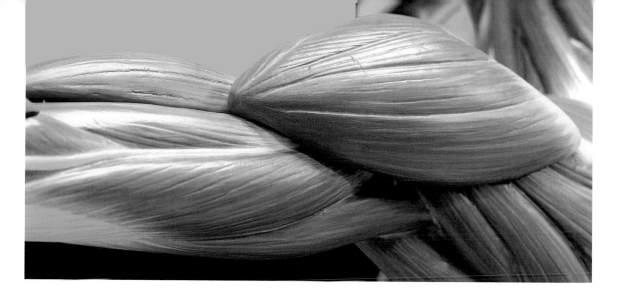

concentrates. The two most common forms are concentrates and isolates, as hydrolysates are more expensive and push up the price of the shake. The main difference is that isolates and hydrolysates are more pure than concentrates, meaning other non-protein components have been partially removed to "isolate" the whey protein.

Concentrates usually consist of about 80% protein, with the remaining 20% of the product made up of carbohydrate (in the form of lactose) and fat. Isolates and hydrolysates are typically about 92% protein. The difference between isolates and hydrolysates is that isolates are available as intact proteins, whereas hydrolysates have been pre-digested, i.e. partially broken down, which should allow them to be absorbed more rapidly. As well as the increased cost of hydrolysates, another disadvantage is that the pre-digested processing can affect the taste, making it bitter. As all three forms are readily digested and absorbed by the body, it is questionable whether the minimally faster digestion rate of hydrolysates is worth the extra money.

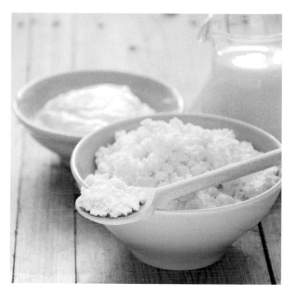

TOP: The muscle structure of the arm.

ABOVE: Dairy products such as cottage cheese are a good source of the branched-chain amino acids that have been shown to be particularly important for protein synthesis.

The bottom line: In terms of convenience and timing, protein shakes do offer a practical solution to recovery from a strenuous workout, but you could just as easily tuck in to a tub of yogurt or cottage cheese to deliver the same amount of protein.

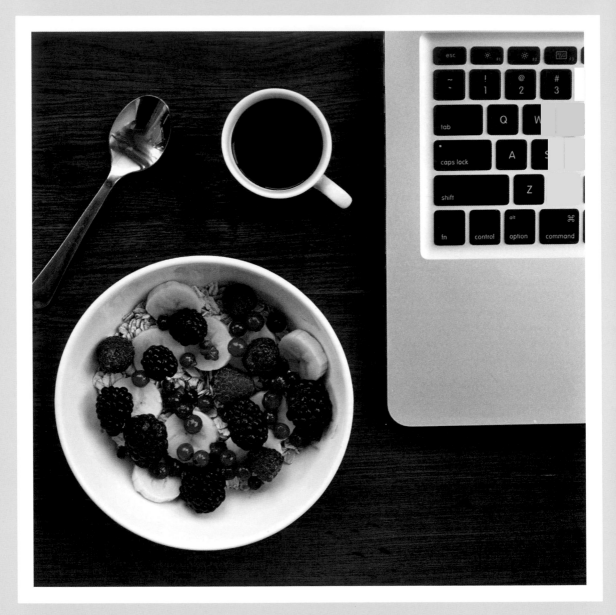

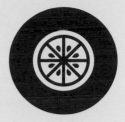

8

THE MOST IMPORTANT MEAL OF THE DAY

Myths relating to breakfast

IS BREAKFAST THE MOST IMPORTANT MEAL OF THE DAY?

Breakfast is generally considered to be a healthy way to start the day, and more important than other meals.

IT IS HARD to disagree when "don't skip breakfast" is part of official government advice on how to eat well and stay healthy. However, the origins of this well-known directive – and indeed the good reputation of breakfast – come from a surprising place.

In 1917 an article appeared in *Good Health* (often credited with being the world's oldest health magazine), which stated that "breakfast is the most important meal of the day, because it is the meal that gets the day started". The editor of the magazine was none other than Dr John Harvey Kellogg, the founder of Kellogg's! It goes on to say that "it should not be eaten hurriedly, and all the family, so far as possible, should partake of it together. And above all, it should be made up of easily digested foods, and balanced in such a way that the various food elements are

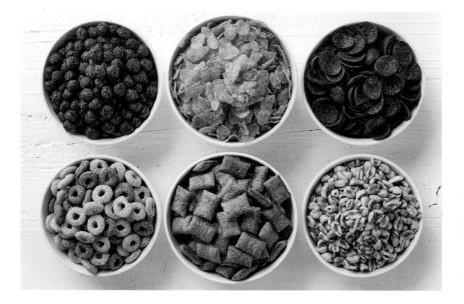

LEFT: Cereal is a popular breakfast, but eggs and yoghurt are probably better choices.

OPPOSITE: It is very easy to snack mindlessly when sitting at a desk.

present in the right proportions. It should not be a heavy meal, consisting of over five to seven hundred calories." The message was a clear swipe at the more traditional choice at that time of eggs and bacon.

"AL DESKO" DINING

There is no doubt that, during the first half of the last century, breakfast would have been a particularly important meal for those who engaged in manual labour, many of whom began working hours before breakfast and would stop to rest and refuel. During the latter decades, eating breakfast remained important as the availability and accessibility of "on the go" food was limited. It was unusual for most people working in factories, institutions or offices to stop for a quick snack when they felt hungry or eat at their desk while they worked.

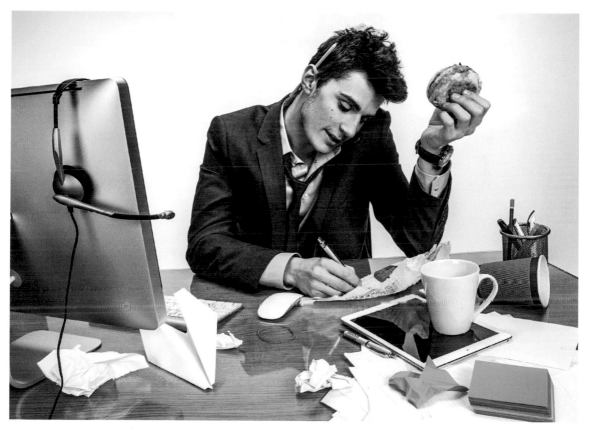

The bottom line: Times have now changed and very few of us need to eat a big bowl of carbohydrates to get us through a strenuous morning tapping on our laptops; most of us have the freedom to eat what we like when we feel like it.

Breakfast does remain an important meal for children and vulnerable individuals who may rely on others to feed them, but in these modern times breakfast is viewed as a choice, depending on how much fuel you need to get you through the morning.

DOES SKIPPING BREAKFAST MAKE YOU FAT?

So many of us find we do not have time for breakfast. In the UK it is thought that as many as one in three people skip breakfast, while in the US this figure is one in ten. It is believed that this could be a key factor in rising obesity rates: breakfast helps us lose weight, we are told, and skipping it causes weight gain. But what's the science behind this counterintuitive claim?

A POPULAR VIEW IS that eating breakfast "kick-starts" metabolism, and an increased metabolic rate means more calories are burned up. Certainly it is true that, whenever a meal is eaten, there is a temporary small but significant increase in metabolic rate known as the thermic effect of food (see page 33). However, this effect is proportional to what is eaten, not when it is eaten. What it doesn't do is set your metabolism off at an increased rate for the rest of the day.

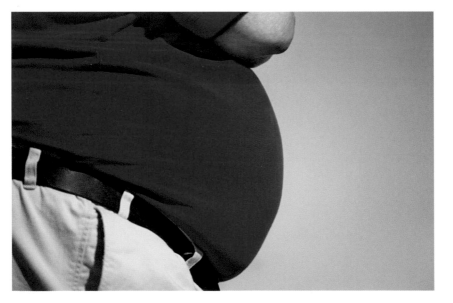

LEFT: *Eating breakfast is not a guarantee of weight loss.*

OPPOSITE ABOVE: *Porridge is a good choice for the busy, but do you need a big bowl of carbohydrates to get you though a morning?*

OPPOSITE BELOW: *Does skipping breakfast really mean you won't be able to control your biscuit craving later on?*

One study that investigated the effect of breakfast-skipping on energy metabolism found that the skipped breakfast was compensated for by having bigger meals at lunch and supper – but made no difference to the total number of calories burned during a 24-hour day.

Then there are claims that people who skip breakfast are also more likely to indulge in an unhealthy mid-morning snack, and put weight on that way. However, recent studies have challenged this, indicating that there is not generally a problem of overcompensation later; in fact, there is evidence to suggest that people who skip breakfast usually consume fewer calories during the day than those who don't skip it.

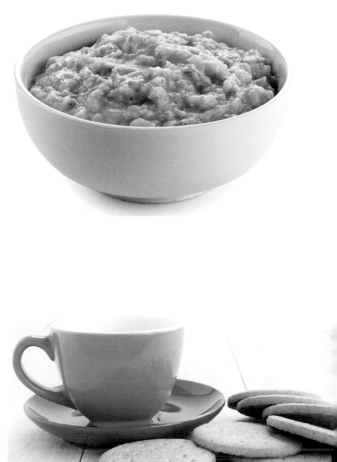

BREAKFAST AND OVERALL HEALTH

Proponents of breakfast claim that breakfast-eaters are healthier overall. This is backed up by many observational studies that show them to have healthier behaviours and a lower risk of chronic conditions such as heart disease and diabetes.

The trouble with observational studies is that they do not demonstrate causation. In other words, these studies show that people who have breakfast are more likely to be healthier, but they cannot prove that the breakfast itself causes this. Breakfast-eaters may be healthier because they follow other wellness advice, such as exercising regularly, not smoking and moderating their salt, fat, sugar and alcohol intake – and because they are not too rushed to eat.

The bottom line: With changing lifestyles, the different ways in which people work and the huge choice of foods we have available to us pretty much 24/7, breakfast should be a choice, not a dictate. Do you need a bowl of porridge to get you through an office meeting? Probably not, but if you don't want to be distracted by hunger, a lighter choice of yogurt or eggs is a good idea. A bowl of porridge is the perfect choice for those spending a morning on their feet in a busy ward, classroom or warehouse. I often work from home and on those mornings I may not eat until I feel hungry at around 11 a.m., but I may well grab some breakfast if I have an early start and don't want to be tempted by pastries with my coffee. With a bit of thought as to what the day ahead holds, where we will be, what we will be doing, we should make our own choices about when we eat our first meal of the day.

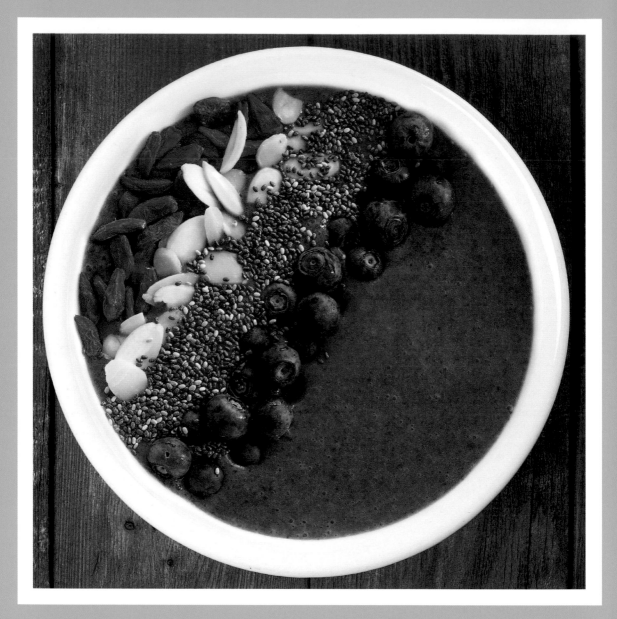

9

SO-CALLED SUPER-FOODS, AND OTHER MYTHS

Myths relating to specific foods and ingredients

ARE SOME FOODS "SUPER"?

What makes a food super? How does an ordinary food or drink become elevated to superstar status? Will regular intake of such superfoods prolong our lives and/or ward off disease?

THE FIRST CHALLENGE ARISES right here at the outset, as there is no agreed scientific or legal definition of what a superfood might be. Neither is there a formula or combination of nutrients or non-nutrients (such as phytochemicals) that must be present. Furthermore, there is no definitive scientific proof that feasting on superfoods will make you live longer or become more beautiful, or protect you against disease. Current European food law states that there is no evidence that blueberries, or antioxidants extracted from them, delay ageing. And so use of the term "superfood",

much loved by the media and food and advertising industries, is all rather subjective, but it makes an attractive marketing piece. A quick search of print and online sources typically provides endless lists of foods deemed to be super: generally specific fruits, vegetables, nuts, seeds or fish. On occasion, oats, quinoa or low-fat yogurts are also promoted to superstardom. More recently, even butter has been added to that list. Sometimes superfoods are described as "nutrient powerhouses", sometimes as "nutrient-dense", other times as "magic bullets" . . . but is there any benefit – or harm – in singling out specific foods?

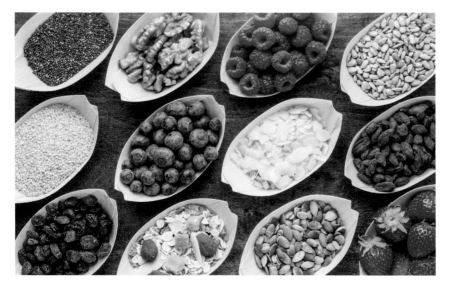

LEFT: Is it right to rank foods? They are all sources of important nutrients.

Will fruit and veg save your life?

Fruit and vegetables are all you need to eat, right? They don't cause cancer or clog you up, they can be eaten raw, and they neutralize acids, make you live longer and cure diseases, don't they? Sadly not: there is no solid scientific evidence to back all this up. True, fruits and vegetables contain lots of vitamins, minerals, fibre, water and phytochemicals, yet provide relatively few calories. They are helpful as part of weight-loss or weight-maintenance regimes, and should be a mainstay of all of our diets. However, they are not always the best sources for certain nutrients – for instance, iron from spinach or goji berries is not absorbed by the body as easily as iron from red meat, and calcium from sesame seeds is not absorbed as readily as that from dairy produce. To obtain the same amount of calcium as there is in a glass of regular milk, you would need to eat around 25 tablespoons of sesame seeds.

Moreover, a fruit-and-vegetable-only diet is not appropriate for someone undergoing cancer treatment, which often triggers weight loss; instead, energy-rich diets, containing fruit and vegetables along with other foods, such as those that provide protein, are needed. And though they contain both carbohydrates and fibre, fruit and vegetables are also not enough for someone who participates in sports or has an active job, or for growing children and teenagers – energy (carbohydrate) is also needed from grains, cereals and roots.

Nutrition aside, including other foods provides taste and variety, and can make social eating easier too!

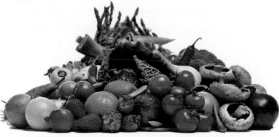

ABOVE: Fruit and veg are important components of a healthy diet, but they cannot deliver everything the body needs.

AVOID EXCESS

The truth is that the foods defined as super are generally healthy in nature. Their consumption fits naturally into a healthy, balanced diet. However, a reasonable degree of scepticism also helps; yes, butter is tasty and made with minimal processing but it is also high in calories and contains a type of fat which, when eaten in excess, can raise cholesterol levels, so excess consumption should be avoided. Also to be avoided is the notion that intake of a specific variety of a food is better than another (e.g. kale is better than regular cabbage or goji berries are better than raspberries) or that specific foods can reduce risk of disease or stop the ageing process. All such foods contain a variety of nutrients – vitamins, minerals and phytochemicals.

The bottom line: It is the combination of foods that we consume that is key to our long-term health and wellbeing, not over-consuming one, two or even a medley of a few foods.

Furthermore, healthy eating need not be expensive. If you choose to buy goji berries, oysters and kale, please enjoy them, but nutritionally you will get similar benefits from cheaper, seasonal alternatives.

ARE VITAMIN WATERS BETTER THAN MINERAL WATERS?

Water with added vitamins and minerals definitely sounds like a good thing. Usually sold with catchy names and in a range of enticing hues, vitamin waters are appealing to the eye and the palate, but are they better for you than regular mineral waters?

THE FIRST THING a savvy shopper must watch out for is the sugar content of such waters. Plain tap water or mineral water does not contain calories. In contrast, some vitamin waters contain sugar, or some form of sugar (be it cane sugar, sucrose, fructose, etc.). The higher up it appears on the ingredient listing, the greater the amount present – and the more calories it will provide. In some instances, the calorie content is comparable to that of regular soft drinks. Care should also be taken with regard to dental health – it is actually best to drink a sugar-containing drink in one go than to sip it at intervals and prolong tooth exposure to caries-causing sugar. Some varieties of vitamin waters contain artificial sweeteners rather than sugar, so this last point becomes less relevant.

ADDED VITAMINS

The interested shopper should then question the vitamins and minerals provided. In general, the vitamins provided are vitamin C or come from the B-vitamin family, all of which are water-soluble. Consuming these waters will boost your intake of these vitamins, but we should remember that our diets typically contain ample amounts of them

already – we are topping up what we naturally consume plenty of, and the body is quite efficient at removing any excess that we don't need. Also present may be minerals such as potassium, magnesium, zinc or chromium, or the fat-soluble

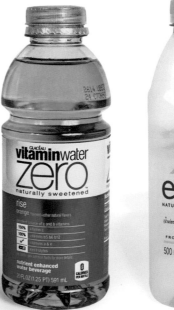
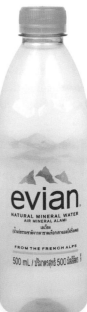

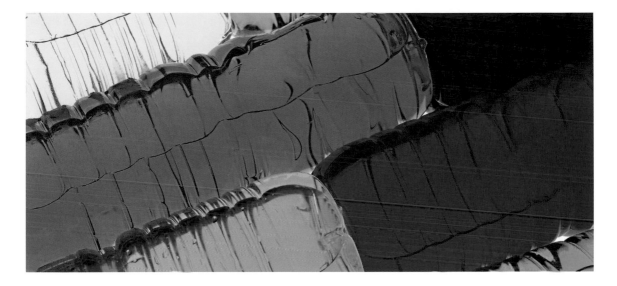

vitamins A and E – of which, again, we generally consume enough already in our diets. But let's not forget that standard mineral water contains minerals too, particularly calcium and magnesium. For the fat-soluble vitamins A and E, fat is also needed to ensure efficient absorption by the body, so drinking the vitamin-containing water in isolation is unlikely to result in good uptake of these fat-soluble vitamins: it is best to consume the water alongside a fat-containing meal.

DOES THE COLOUR MATTER?

Eyebrows may be raised at the bright colours of the waters, the use of processes such as "reverse osmosis", or the inclusion of ingredients such as caffeine or taurine. To a large degree, these are all just gimmicks. Some consumers may be reassured to read on packaging that the colours and flavours used are "natural". However, even use of artificial colours or flavours should pose no risk to health – any used will have been deemed safe for consumption by the European Food Safety Authority or its equivalents worldwide. Reverse osmosis is just a purification step used to remove particles of various sizes from drinking water. It's typically used in laboratory experiments sensitive to the presence of molecules or ions, but there's no advantage for human health. Our bodies are perfectly equipped – and indeed designed – to deal with such molecules or ions. In any case, molecules and ions are added back into these beverages with the inclusion of sugars or sweeteners, vitamins, minerals and flavours. Caffeine and/or taurine may be added for purported stimulant properties, but again there's no added advantage to health.

....

OPPOSITE: Minerals are naturally present in spring water, whereas vitamins have to be added.

ABOVE: It is not the addition of vitamins that gives these bottled waters their attractive hues, but food-colour additives.

The bottom line: Relative to standard mineral waters, there is no added benefit from consuming vitamin waters. It comes back again to personal preference – and how deep your purse is.

DOES SOYA PREVENT THE MENOPAUSE?... AND OTHER MIRACLES

Soya frequently appears in the media under conflicting headlines; it might be the answer to the menopause or it might turn my son into a daughter. What exactly is soya, and are any of these claims valid?

IT HAS BEEN INVESTIGATED for its effect on many different conditions, from heart disease to cancer, and more than 2,000 soya-related peer-reviewed articles are published annually. The results from trials and studies are far from uniform and it is often difficult to interpret the evidence into meaningful and practical guidance on how much soya to eat – or indeed whether or not to eat soya at all.

NUTRITIONAL COMPOSITION OF SOYA

Soya beans are classified as a legume. However, their nutrient composition differs markedly from other legumes: it is much higher in fat, moderately higher in protein and much lower in carbohydrate.

Not only do soya beans have a higher total protein content than other beans, but the quality of soya protein is also superior to that of other plant proteins; in fact, it is similar to animal protein. Quality of protein is determined by a DIAAS (digestible indispensable amino

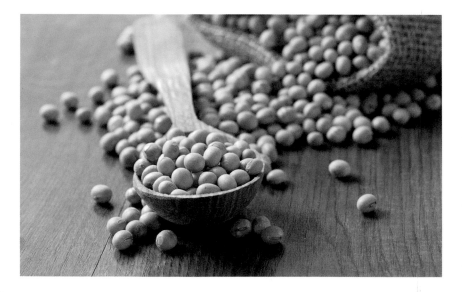

LEFT: There has been a huge amount of research into the potential health benefits and disadvantages of soya beans.

OPPOSITE ABOVE: Soya beans are used to make a variety of products including milks, tofu and tempeh.

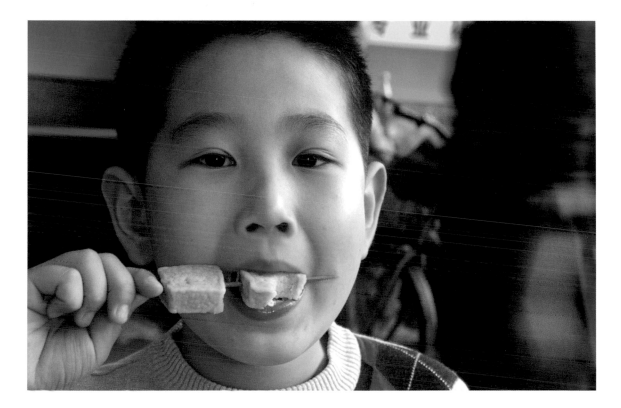

acid score) value. This is a measure of the quantity of essential amino acids a protein contains. Essential amino acids cannot be made in the body and thus it is necessary to consume them in the diet. The DIAAS value for soya protein is 0.9, which is well above the minimum value of 0.75 that defines high-quality protein.

Soya beans are high in fibre and low in carbohydrate. They contain a type of carbohydrate known as oligosaccharides, which are poorly digested by intestinal enzymes and so pass through to the colon, where they are able to stimulate the growth of friendly bacteria such as bifidobacteria, meaning soya-bean oligosaccharides are classified as prebiotics.

The fat content of soya beans varies between different varieties, but generally they are low in saturated fat and high in polyunsaturated fat. Their polyunsaturated fat content is made up of the essential fatty acids linoleic acid and alpha-linolenic acid in a fairly equal ratio. This equal ratio is unusual in foods and makes the soya bean quite unique in being a good source of both essential fatty acids.

The soya bean is a good source of a variety of vitamins and minerals, including calcium and iron. The absorption of calcium and iron from soya is an important consideration because soya foods often replace foods that are good sources of these minerals, such as milk and meat. When it comes to iron, soya is usually thought of as a poor replacement for meat, since iron from non-meat sources is less well absorbed, but relatively new research shows iron absorption from soya is better than previously assumed.

Aside from the impressive nutrient content of soya, most of the research interest stems from its isoflavones.

Isoflavones are naturally occurring compounds found in many different plant foods, but soya beans are a particularly rich source. There are three main isoflavones, namely genistein, daidzein and glycitein, and these account for approximately 50%, 40% and 10% respectively of the total isoflavone content of soya beans. Each gram of soya protein is associated with approximately 3.5mg of isoflavones. This means 100g (3.5oz) of tofu (made from mashed soya beans) or 250ml (8.5fl oz) of soya milk provides about 25mg of isoflavones. In more processed products, such as protein shakes that use isolated soya protein, as much as 80–90% of the isoflavone content can be lost as a result of processing.

There is a huge difference in consumption of isoflavones around the world. In some Asian countries where soya beans are a staple, such as Japan, intake may range from 30 to 50mg per day, compared with less than 3mg per day in the United States, Canada and Europe.

Most of the interest in isoflavones lies in the fact that they are phytoestrogens – this means they have a chemical structure similar to the hormone oestrogen, which allows them to bind to oestrogen receptors in the body and produce oestrogen-like effects in certain conditions.

The conflicting results presented in the peer reviews mentioned earlier are due to many confounding issues. Many of the studies have been conducted on mice and rats, but it is known that they metabolize isoflavones differently to humans. There is also a striking difference in isoflavone metabolism among humans. Only about 25% of non-Asians and 50% of Asians have the ability to convert isoflavones into their active form (where they are able to act as a phytoestrogens). This leads to the hypothesis that only some people could actually benefit from soya beans.

DOES SOYA PROTECT AGAINST HEART DISEASE?

Research has shown that a regular intake of 25g (0.9oz) or more of soya per day can help to lower

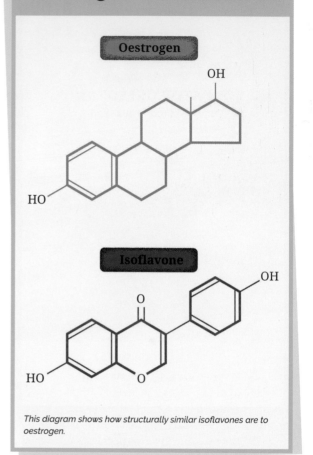

Oestrogen and isoflavone

This diagram shows how structurally similar isoflavones are to oestrogen.

LDL or "bad" cholesterol in the blood. Raised LDL-cholesterol has been associated with an increased risk of heart disease. However, this is a big dose and is more soya protein than would be eaten even by many people living in Asian countries eating a traditional diet. It is unlikely that this dose could be consumed in the context of a Western diet without making huge changes. To achieve this in a day, you would have to consume 250ml of soya milk (maybe half on cereal, the rest in drinks), 75g (2.6oz) of tofu or soya mince and a soya yogurt. Confounding the problem of daily quantity further is the fact that about 20% of individuals whose cholesterol levels are raised do not respond to dietary changes. So often the effects achieved with soya protein are rather modest and may not be much different from those achieved by adopting a healthier diet and lifestyle in general.

DOES SOYA STOP OSTEOPOROSIS?

The onset of the menopause brings changes in hormone levels and in particular a drop in the level of oestrogen in the body. Bones become weaker with age but with a lack of oestrogen comes an acceleration of loss of bone mass and an increased risk of osteoporosis (brittleness) and bone fracture. Given the ability of the phytoestrogens in soya to mimic the effects of oestrogen in the body, it has been suggested that consumption of soya could reduce the rate of bone-mass decline and protect bone health.

This was supported by the results from two large studies in Asian women, which found that soya intake was associated with a one-third reduction in fracture risk. However, as part of a traditional diet, their soya intake may just be a marker for an overall healthy diet that provides other nutrients important for bone health. Many short-term studies have found that isoflavones have a positive effect on the bone health of post-menopausal women, but to date the larger, long-term studies have shown disappointing results in the ability of soya to promote bone health over other foods that contain high-quality protein and well-absorbed calcium, such as dairy products.

BELOW: A normal human spine (left) compared to the spine of a patient who has osteoporosis (right).

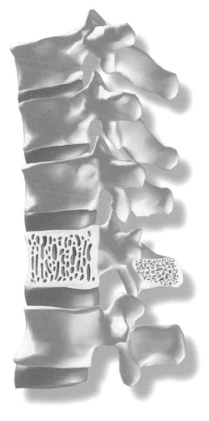
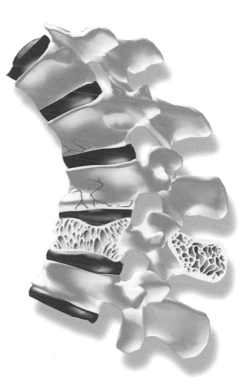

DOES SOYA REDUCE RISK OF BREAST CANCER?

Global rates of breast cancer differ significantly between Asian and Western countries, leading to the hypothesis that consuming soya could protect against breast cancer. This hypothesis is strengthened by the fact that a rise in breast cancer has been observed in some sectors of the Asian population where the diet has become more Westernized and therefore contains less soya. Once again, the protective effects of the soya are thought to be from the isoflavones and their ability to regulate the levels of oestrogen in the body. However, most studies show that, for soya to reduce risk, its consumption must start early and be consumed regularly during childhood and adolescence. In Western countries this is generally a marker of good health and, as studies using soya supplements do not demonstrate a protective effect, it is more likely that a healthy diet and lifestyle from an early age is really what protects against breast cancer.

SHOULD WOMEN RECOVERING FROM BREAST CANCER AVOID EATING SOYA?

Oestrogen has been found to stimulate breast-cancer cells and cause an existing tumour to grow. Therefore it has been suggested that women with breast cancer or who have recovered from breast cancer should avoid eating soya as the phytoestrogens will act like oestrogen in the body. However, most of the studies that have shown that phytoestrogens increase the growth of a breast-cancer tumour have been conducted in mice. Rodents metabolize isoflavones differently from humans, so the value of these studies for understanding effects in humans is in doubt.

More recent data has shown that soya isoflavones, even in large doses, do not exert harmful effects on breast tissue. The European Food Safety Authority has concluded that neither soya nor isoflavone supplements affect breast-cancer prognosis.

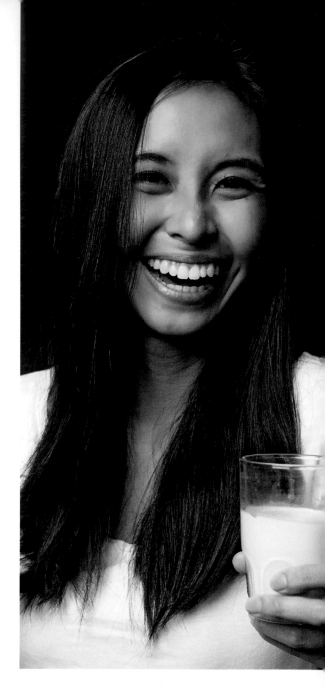

ABOVE: Soya milk, which originated in China, is made by soaking, grinding and boiling dried soya beans.

OPPOSITE ABOVE: It is unlikely that soya consumption can prevent wrinkles, however much we would like it to be the case.

DOES SOYA PREVENT THE MENOPAUSE?

Hot flashes are the most common reason given by women seeking treatment for menopausal symptoms. The low prevalence of hot flashes among native Japanese women, combined with the knowledge that isoflavones interact with oestrogen receptors, has led to the hypothesis that soya foods prevent the onset of hot flashes and could be capable of alleviating existing hot flashes. The first trial to test this hypothesis was published in the early 1990s. Since then, at least 25 trials have evaluated the effects of a variety of soya products on menopause-related hot flashes and have produced inconsistent results.

DOES SOYA PREVENT WRINKLES?

The impact of soya, and more specifically isoflavones, on skin health including wrinkles, is another area of great interest. Isoflavones bind to oestrogen receptors, which are present in the skin, and because oestrogen therapy is thought to improve a number of skin conditions it is hoped that isoflavones could do the same. Several trials have suggested that isoflavones help to reduce wrinkles but on closer inspection, these trials have been heavily criticized in their design and interpretation of the results.

DOES SOYA BRING EARLY PUBERTY?

With puberty occurring at an ever-earlier age, soya has been identified as a possible culprit due to the ability of phytoestrogens to act like oestrogen. This

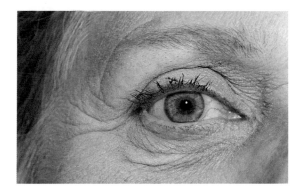

has led to concern about the possible hormonal effects of soya consumption in children. Few studies have investigated this issue and, so far, the evidence suggests neither soya nor isoflavones affect hormone levels in childhood and bring on early puberty. Many other factors can affect early puberty, including increasing weight and protein consumption, both of which are far more pertinent problems today.

DOES SOYA FEMINIZE MEN?

Although there have been case reports describing feminizing effects that allegedly occurred as a result of soya consumption, the individuals involved were said to have consumed 360mg per day of isoflavones, which is nine times greater than the average intake among older Japanese men eating a traditional (i.e. soya-heavy) diet. In the context of such unbalanced and probably nutrient-deficient diets, it is difficult to conclude the true impact of the isoflavones.

The bottom line: Soya foods can be enjoyed as part of a healthy, balanced diet. They do not need to replace existing healthy foods, but rather add variety. Their versatility allows them to be incorporated easily and provides a convenient way to exploit the nutritional advantages of legumes, such as their higher protein and fibre content, healthy fatty-acid profile and good amounts of well-absorbed minerals. When adding soya to the diet it is important to consider the overall nutritional quality of a particular soya food since many processed soya foods could be full of sugar. Ideally, soya foods should be incorporated into the diet by displacing less healthy foods, such as swapping a fizzy drink for a glass of soya milk.

WILL SWEETENERS HELP YOU LOSE WEIGHT?

Any product that is low in calories can help aid weight loss, right? Although often believed to be a "new" ingredient, the first artificial sweetener (saccharin) was actually discovered in 1879 at Johns Hopkins University in the United States.

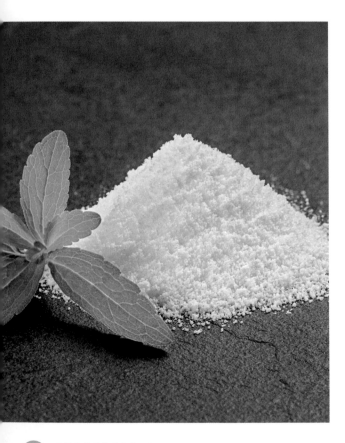

HOWEVER, WIDESPREAD USE BEGAN in the 1980s, and sweeteners now appear under a variety of names, among them saccharin, sucralose, steviol glycosides, aspartame, cyclamate, neotame and acesulfame potassium. All are approved as safe to consume in Europe.

By their nature, sweeteners – sometimes called low-calorie or non-nutritive sweeteners – are low in calories (usually 0–4kcal/g) but impart much greater sweetening power compared to pure sugar (sucrose), so only tiny amounts need be used. Differences in sweetening power can range from 30 times sweeter than sugar for cyclamate, to up to 13,000 times sweeter than sugar for neotame. Artificial sweeteners are typically added to foods usually associated with a high-calorie or high-sugar content (e.g. soft drinks, desserts, dairy products, confectionery, hot chocolate drinks, breakfast cereals). So is it reasonable to assume that substitution of sugar with such sweeteners will yield lower-calorie options and aid weight loss?

LEFT: Steviol glycosides, found in stevia, are 150 times sweeter than sugar.

VARIETY IS SWEET

The answer is not so clear-cut. Yes, added to single foods, they will of course reduce the calorie content. They can also improve palatability and when used as blends (to resemble sugar) mean that high levels of sweetness can be imparted using relatively low amounts. Inclusion of artificially sweetened foods in a diet plan can also add variety and choice and help ensure diet adherence and success, not only during the dieting phase but also when trying to keep the lost weight from piling back on again – the so-called weight-maintenance phase. They do not negatively affect dental health. However, it is important to bear in mind that it is the sum total of dietary intake (and accompanying levels of physical [in]activity) that will determine whether weight is lost or gained. Switch your regular soda to a diet soda and you will automatically reduce calorie intake, but if you compensate for those "saved" calories elsewhere in your diet, weight will not be lost.

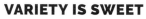

ABOVE: Replacing sugar in hot drinks with sweeteners can reduce calorie intake.

RIGHT: Diet drinks outsell their sugary counterparts.

The bottom line: Given that weight gain arises for a number of reasons, simply switching to artificial sweeteners is unlikely to be a successful strategy for losing weight on its own, but it may help. One thing is sure: given the intense scrutiny on sugar, particularly added sugar intake, it is likely that food manufacturers will increasingly rely on artificial sweeteners to impart sweetness.

IS COCONUT WATER MORE HYDRATING THAN WATER?

At my local gym there is a floor-to-ceiling poster recommending coconut water for your post-workout means of rehydration. And I have certainly noticed more people carrying a carton of coconut water into class rather than a bottle of water. So are all these people on to something or have they just been taking in by clever marketing?

THE INTEREST IN COCONUT water as a means of providing effective hydration lies in that fact that its composition is similar to that of isotonic sports drinks. Coconut water comes from the inside of a coconut and contains about 18 calories, 4.5g of carbohydrates (3.6g as natural sugars), 28mg of sodium and almost 200mg of potassium per 100ml. In comparison, plain bottled water has no calories, carbohydrates, sodium or potassium. The nutrient profile of an isotonic sports drink varies among brands but, on average, 100ml will provide 24 calories, 6g of carbohydrates (all in the form of added sugar), 42mg of sodium and 12mg of potassium.

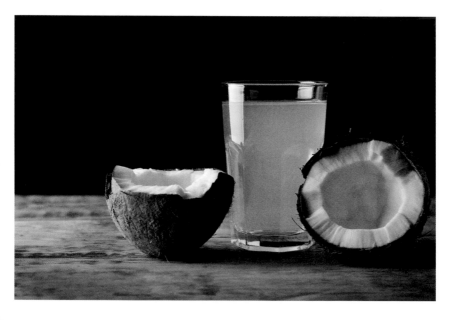

LEFT: Coconut water is growing in popularity as the choice of drink for exercise.

OPPOSITE LEFT: For most people water is just as good a choice.

OPPOSITE RIGHT: Coconut water may be more palatable than other formulated sports drinks.

Isotonic drinks are designed to have salt and sugar concentrations similar to those found in body cells, and this increases the rate at which water can pass into the body. They are thought to have the fastest rates of absorption and so can be useful during exercise when quick replacement of fluid, salts and energy is needed. But there is little advantage in a fast rate of rehydration after exercise has finished; the water from any drink will be absorbed as the body needs it.

COCONUT WATER AFTER EXERCISE

Only a few studies have looked at the impact of coconut water on rehydration after exercise, the majority of them reporting little to no difference between coconut water, traditional sports drinks and water.

Studies comparing the effects of coconut water, coconut water from concentrate, bottled water and sports drinks on rehydration found that the water provided similar rehydrating effects to both coconut waters (fresh and from concentrate) and the sports drink.

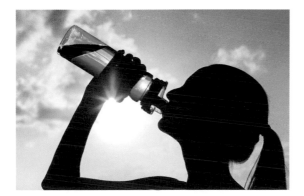

COCONUT AFTER ENDURANCE

However, the researchers did report one advantage of the coconut water, in that it seemed to cause less nausea and fullness, and no stomach upset. An upset tummy can be a common complaint from participants in endurance events such as marathons. Rehydration is recommended as part of recovery, but many people do not feel like eating or drinking soon after finishing. In the studies, the coconut water was easier to consume in larger amounts compared to both plain water and the sports drink.

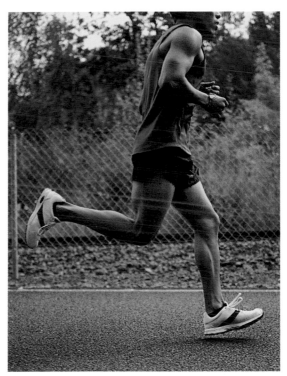

The bottom line: As far as hydration goes, the evidence suggests that, when consumed in adequate quantities, plain water, coconut water and sports drinks are all comparable. For the majority of people, who are exercising in order to lose or maintain a healthy weight and who work out for 60 minutes or less under normal conditions (i.e. not in extreme heat and humidity), water remains the best and most affordable choice.

DO FAT-BURNING FOODS BURN MORE CALORIES?

Of all of the potential "wonder foods", surely a food that could burn fat would be the Holy Grail?

A QUICK SEARCH OF the Internet will yield any number of sites suggesting that you can "rev up your metabolism" or "burn more calories" by choosing from an array of foods, typically including peppers, chillies, whole grains (particularly oats), certain fruits and vegetables, teas and some oily fish. (Don't they sound remarkably like the superfood list?) The rationale ranges from staving off hunger and keeping you full for longer (in the case of oats) to stimulating production of hormones relating to appetite (leptin) and glucose uptake by the body (insulin), as well as simply "boosting metabolic rate".

BELOW LEFT: Oats provide slow-release energy, which helps you exercise for longer and burn more calories.

BELOW RIGHT: Green tea contains caffeine, which temporarily boosts your metabolic rate.

OPPOSITE: How spicy can you take your food? The more chilli you add the more calories you will burn.

....

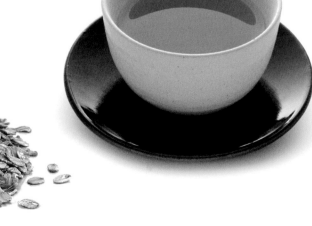

The power of chillies

There have been some interesting studies on the potential of chillies to aid weight loss. Experiments in animals and humans have shown that consuming a meal containing chilli increases energy expenditure and fat oxidation compared to the same meal without chilli. This has led to the suggestion that regular chilli consumption could help reduce obesity. However, there are drawbacks: not everyone relishes the thought of a spicy breakfast and for some people spicy food can cause unpleasant and embarrassing side effects. The amount of chilli required for it to have an effect is high – some studies have used a 30g per day dose. Furthermore, the effect could be lost over time as the body adapts to this intake. If you like chilli, there is no harm in consuming a little more but don't expect miraculous results and don't use it as an excuse to eat unhealthy food. In other words, a hotter curry does not mean a cake later.

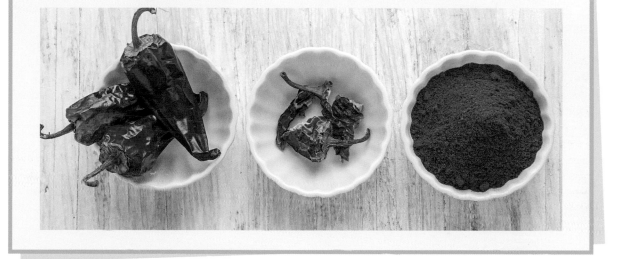

DOES IT WORK?

However, nice as it sounds, there is no solid evidence that any food or drinks are "fat burning" or "burn more calories" (see also page 38). There is no approved link in Europe or the US between any of these foods and burning calories. A quick glance at the above list would suggest that most of these foods are not calorie-laden in their pure form and most contain lots of regular nutrients – so they can form part of healthy, balanced diets, but they don't burn more calories per se. While there is some scientific research trying to ascertain whether green-tea extracts can influence fat mass and weight loss, at present there is no solid proof that consumption of green-tea extracts will burn fat or improve weight loss in humans to any meaningful degree.

The bottom line: As ever, it is the totality of our food intake and the amount of energy we burn off that dictates our body size.

DO YOU NEED SALT IN YOUR DIET?

Depending on your viewpoint, salt is either a tasty addition to the diet or one of the biggest contributors to ill health and to conditions such as high blood pressure and strokes.

GOVERNMENTS WORLDWIDE, including the UK, have established limits on the amount of salt we should consume in our diets, with a maximal value of 6g/day (0.21oz) listed for adults, and lower values for younger age groups. We currently consume around 8g/day (0.28oz). But if less is more, should we be aiming for just 1g (0.035oz), or even 0g, per day?

The truth is that excess salt intake has been associated with an increased likelihood of high blood pressure and stroke. However, we are not all at equal risk: it is greater for some genetically susceptible people than others and for some ethnic groups (e.g. African Caribbean) than others. On the other hand, some sportspeople may require more salt to replace that lost through sweating. We also need to eat salt, or more specifically sodium, as it helps maintain fluid balance in our bodies and also helps nerves and muscles work. In many countries, salt is seen as a vehicle to provide dietary iodine and prevent against iodine-deficiency disease and goitres (swelling of the thyroid gland). From a nutritional point of view, however, we only need around 1g/day of salt, with all salt having similar biological effects irrespective of whether it is common table salt or rock, pink, sea or Himalayan.

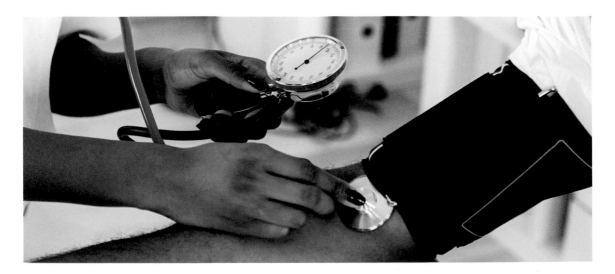

TRUST ME, I'M A DIETICIAN
Alternative ways to flavour your food

Reducing the amount of salt you consume is a bit like giving up sugar in your tea: it takes a bit of getting used to but after a while you are unlikely to miss it. If you want to reduce your salt intake, don't be fooled by gourmet options like sea-salt crystals or Himalayan rock salt: salt is salt and these varieties do not contain less sodium. Similarly celery salt and garlic salt are mainly salt with a little of the dried vegetable added. Blends of salts that contain potassium chloride do contain a lot less sodium but will not help to reduce your taste for salt. If it's seasoning you're craving, then salt is not the only way to flavour your food – there are plenty of alternatives. Try experimenting with herbs and spices, lemon juice, vinegars and infused oils to jazz up your dishes. Persevere and you won't feel the need to reach for the salt.

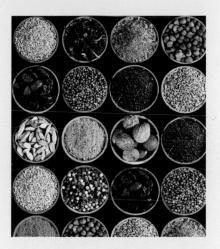

THE CONTRIBUTION OF SALT

The tricky thing with salt is that most of the salt we consume – about 75% – is already contained in our food, so simply avoiding the salt cellar won't eliminate salt from your diet. But let's not forget that salt makes an important contribution to food. It preserves meats and pickles and helps avoid food spoilage by keeping food safe to eat for longer. Adding salt during bread-making is also necessary to strengthen the dough and to influence the fermentation rate. During manufacture of breakfast cereals, salt affects colour and taste. Across the board, salt provides flavour.

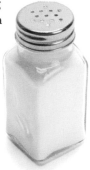

OPPOSITE: For some people, blood-pressure readings are raised by prolonged excess salt intake.

ABOVE: Experiment with herbs and spices to add flavour to your food.

RIGHT: To lower your salt intake, taste your food before automatically adding salt at the table.

The bottom line: So should we remove salt from our diet? In theory we could, but in practice it would be very hard and not necessary. Over the last 10 years there have been a series of initiatives by governments and the food industry to reduce the salt content of foods we consume before they even reach the table. We can further reduce our salt intake by cutting back on salt added at the table or in cooking, or by using peppers and spices for taste instead. You don't need to remove salt from your diet, but you can take practical steps to avoid excessive intake (see also page 129).

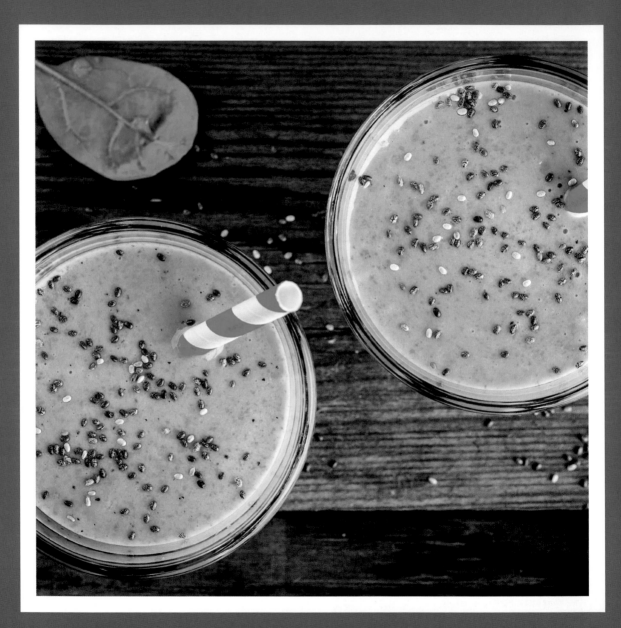

10

ON-TREND EATING

Myths relating to diet fads

WELCOME TO THE DIET CULT

Fad diets make the headlines and grab our attention because we can't resist the promise of a quick-fix weight-loss/health gain and we are bored with hearing that weight loss is only achieved through a sensible, slow, long-term approach.

FOR MOST OF US, the greatest hurdle in weight loss is keeping the weight off – fad diets get everyone excited because they can promote fast results, but most people tire of the regimes and restrictions and put the weight back on. This yo-yo effect is not only demoralizing for the individual but also bad for the body. Research shows that people who attempt to lose a small amount of weight each week (1–2lb, or 0.5–1kg) by following a healthier lifestyle rather than aiming for drastic weight loss by a fad diet are more likely to have maintained a weight reduction one year on.

We have been bombarded with thousands of fad diets over the past 20 years, often popularized by celebrities with enticing claims that are not always true. Along with whole-diet fads, there are crazes concerning specific groups of foods and nutrients, many of which are also inaccurately promoted. In this chapter, let's look at some common fads and misconceptions in the diet arena.

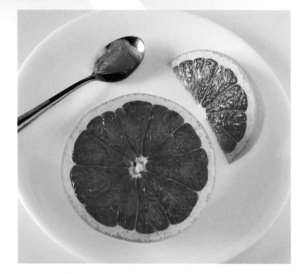

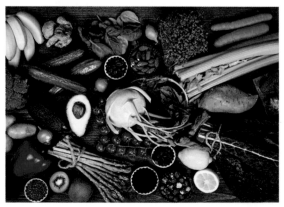

ABOVE RIGHT: The grapefruit diet was a popular fad diet that originated in the 1930s.

RIGHT: Most fad diets are based on the exclusion of one or more food groups.

SHOULD YOU AVOID PROCESSED FOODS?

The proposed benefits of a diet devoid of processed foods range from the avoidance of food chemicals (e.g. artificial sweeteners) to being free of the "additive nature" of processed foods, to increased health and vitality.

PARTICULAR EMPHASIS is usually given to foods containing ingredients such as fat, saturated fat, added sugar, high-fructose corn starch or trans fat.

WHAT IS A PROCESSED FOOD?

Many people misuse the term "processed food", leading to confusion and misinformation. Nearly all food and drinks are in fact processed in some way, by which I mean they are altered from their natural state by various methods, such as heating, salting, canning, fermenting, freezing and so on. These processes have evolved in order to make foods more accessible, convenient and palatable, and sometimes even safer. A simple bread is made by following a recipe (flour, water, salt, yeast, oil) and then baking. Even without the addition of more complex ingredients, e.g. improvers or raising agents, the simple act of mixing and baking is processing. For example, in the UK, US, Canada and Australia, certain vitamins and minerals (e.g. thiamine, niacin and iron) are added to white bread to restore losses that occur during the milling of the grain. This simple restorative measure is also processing, yet it results in increased dietary intakes of these nutrients in the population, since bread is a popular food.

In a similar manner, milk is a processed food – it is pasteurized (to ensure safety) and homogenized (to disperse milk-fat globules and avoid cream rising to the surface).

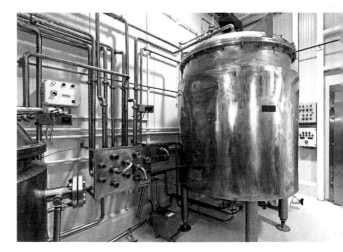

ABOVE: Pasteurization is a form of processing.

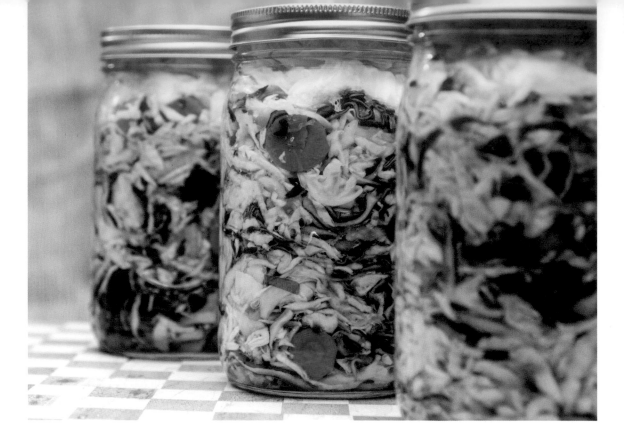

In the UK, milk contributes around 26% to the population's daily dietary calcium intake, while bread contributes approximately 14% to the daily intake of thiamine.

GOOD AND BAD PROCESSING

When discussing processed-food intakes and health, it is useful to classify processed foods according to their degree of processing. The first group may contain minimally processed products: ready-prepared foods such as chopped veggies and frozen, pasteurized and canned foods. These tend to be whole foods, which have undergone some sort of process that doesn't significantly alter their nutritional content. The second group, medium-processed foods, refers to oils, butter, flour and sugar, which are used as ingredients to make the third group, ultra-processed foods. This includes biscuits, bread, cereal, chocolate, sugary drinks, hot dogs, burgers and ready meals.

Many processed foods, particularly from the first group, are an essential convenience to time-poor families and can be a healthy choice. Frozen vegetables and fruits are often processed within hours of being picked so that hardly any nutrients are lost, and they can therefore be considered healthy choices. Processing also turns some otherwise inedible foods into palatable forms; for example, wheat on its own is pretty indigestible but through milling and refining is made into flour and then breads, a staple food for people all over the world.

Ultra-processed foods include foods that have come a long way from their natural state and which often have a lower nutritional content owing to heat exposure or removal of the nutritional portion. They tend to be energy-dense, containing a high number of calories thanks to the addition of sugars and fats, and may contain other additional ingredients such as salt, artificial sweeteners, additives and preservatives. Many people have a fear of food chemicals or artificial ingredients – fear of the unknown, or "nasties" – but any food chemical used in food produced in Europe has been rigorously assessed and then approved for use. The "E" in E numbers simply stands for "Europe", and while this scientific-sounding system may make ingredients sound alien, E300 or ascorbic acid is simply vitamin C, while E308 or gamma tocopherol is vitamin E.

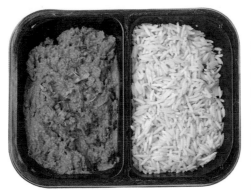

Processing can alter the nature of the food unfavourably, too, for example by increasing its glycaemic index. Such foods have increased dramatically in production and consumption in the past few decades, and it is often this group that people are referring to when they state that processed foods are bad for us. Current government advice suggests individuals should carefully consider their intake of these ultra-processed foods, minimizing quantity, but the reality is that they don't need to be totally avoided because there are nutritious ultra-processed options available. Balanced intakes and knowledge of ingredients are key: look out for hidden sugar, salt and fat. It is estimated that as much as three quarters of our salt intake comes from processed foods, so low-sodium or reduced-salt options are advised.

OPPOSITE: Some foods are processed by fermentation in order to preserve them.

ABOVE: Always check the label to see what has been added to your ready meal.

BELOW LEFT: Sweets may contain an array of artificial ingredients, but these are unlikely to cause you any harm.

BELOW RIGHT: Wheat is processed in order to produce the flour required to make bread.

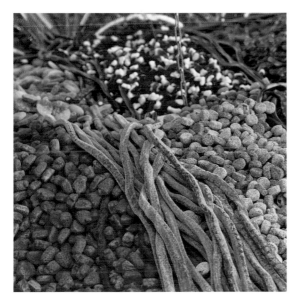

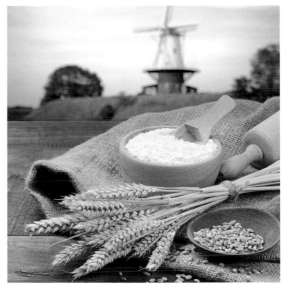

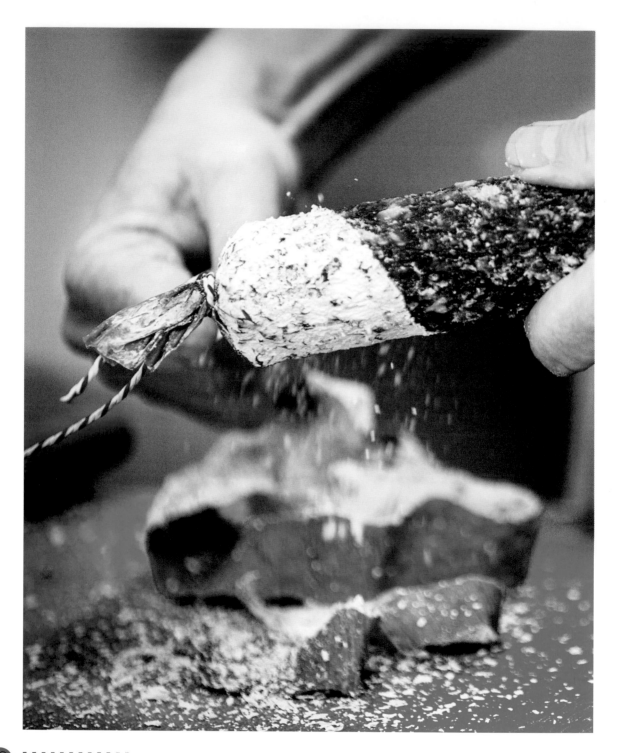

Types of processed foods

Unprocessed	Minimally processed	Processed	Highly processed
Raw fruit	Pure juice	Butter	Ready meals
Raw veg	Wholegrains	Oils	Sauces
Eggs	Milk	Frozen veg	Cereals
Meat	Roasted nuts	Canned beans	Biscuits
Poultry	Bagged salads	Sugar	Sweets
Fish	Prepared fruit	Syrups	Soft drinks
Nuts	Coffee beans	Pasta	Noodle pots
Seeds	Dried beans	Bread	Crackers
Honey	Smoked fish	White rice	Dips

PROCESSED MEATS AND CANCER

There is compelling evidence from the scientific community associating a high intake of some processed meats with an increased risk of bowel cancer. Eating processed meat such as sausages, ham, bacon, salami and pâté can cause damage to DNA in cells; also the method of preserving these meats by salting, smoking or curing may introduce cancer-causing substances. People at risk are those eating more than 90g (3oz) every day (which is equivalent to approximately four or five rashers of back bacon, three thick slices of ham or two sausages). This emphasizes the need for balance in the diet; individuals can make easy substitutes for processed meats to avoid eating them every day, for instance switching a ham sandwich for a tuna sandwich.

We know that increased consumption of ultra-processed foods is associated with poorer health,

namely increased tendency of over-consumption leading to risk of obesity and type 2 diabetes. This group of foods and drinks should not feature heavily in an individual's diet, but including a range of lightly processed foods in the diet is not associated with negative health consequences. We need to be equipped with the knowledge to spot a decent processed food rather than demonizing the whole category.

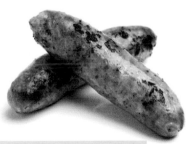

OPPOSITE: Processed red meats include sausages, ham, bacon, salami and pâté.

RIGHT: Consuming a lot of processed red-meat products is linked with increased risk of cancer.

The bottom line: Remove processed foods from your diet if you wish, but you may find your diet very restricted and, more importantly, you may have to look elsewhere to obtain enough nutrients to satisfy your body's needs.

SHOULD YOU EAT LIKE A CAVEMAN?

Diets that suggest eating like a caveman – Stone Age or Palaeolithic diets – are popular with many.

MOST INVOLVE ITERATIONS OF high-protein diets consisting of meat, fish, eggs, some nuts, seeds, fresh fruits and vegetables and select oils. There is no room for carbohydrate-rich foods, most oils and dairy produce. Some versions involve eating little or nothing during the day and feasting in the evening – akin to cavemen coming back to their caves at night. But do they work? And if so, what's the harm?

HUNT FOR THE LOST NUTRIENTS

As with any diet, if you eat fewer calories than you are used to, you will lose weight. It does not matter what the source of the calories is. In the case of caveman diets, it is typically as a result of removing carbohydrates. However, excluding entire food groups from your diet is not advisable in the longer term and may lead you to miss out on key nutrients that your body needs to function and ward off diseases. By cutting out carbohydrates, you remove not only a key source of energy – particularly glucose, which is the brain's preferred fuel – but also fibre, which is needed to keep bowel habits healthy. Cutting out dairy produce removes key sources of calcium, which is needed to maintain bone health and may also protect against high blood pressure. So if you plan to remove these foods from your diet in the longer term, it is best to look for alternative sources, most likely supplements.

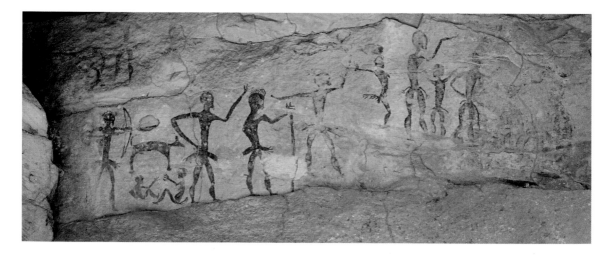

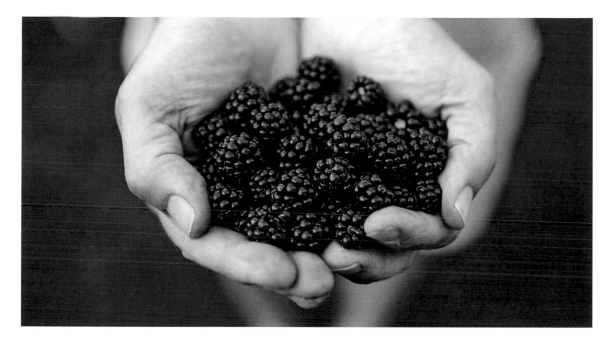

WATCH THE PROTEIN

Other difficulties arise if you consume large amounts of protein sources that are high in fat and saturated fat (e.g. burgers, sausages and other processed meats), as this can raise your cholesterol level and increase your risk of heart disease as well as bowel cancer. Contrary to public perception, there is no firm evidence that such diets improve long-term blood-glucose control – if anything, long-term fasting with irregular meals can be unhelpful in keeping blood-sugar levels within a healthy range. Furthermore, while protein is an important fuel for sport, evidence suggests that protein and carbohydrate are helpful in refuelling post-exercise – protein alone is not enough. For individuals with impaired kidney function in particular, such high protein intakes are not recommended.

OPPOSITE: Cave-painting evidence of our hunter-gather heritage.

ABOVE: Cavemen would have been drawn to the natural sweetness of berries.

BELOW: Consuming a lot of red meat can increase your intake of saturated fat.

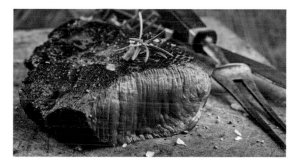

The bottom line: As a short-term weight-loss strategy, following any diet containing fewer calories than usual will of course work. However, there are no advantages of "eating like a caveman", and as the longer-term health effects of such a diet are unknown, it is most likely inadvisable to follow it.

IS RAW FOOD BETTER FOR YOU?

Another diet fad recommends against heating food above 48°C (118°F): the so-called raw-food diet. Some variants of this diet additionally suggest selecting only organic foods (with no preservatives, pesticides or GM organisms) that are as fresh or "wild" as possible.

THE JUSTIFICATION BEHIND THIS diet is that cooking foods supposedly forces your body to work harder – either by making it produce enzymes to digest cooked food or by making the body more acidic in nature and therefore susceptible to disease. In some instances, cooking is also credited with making it harder for your body to absorb nutrients (e.g. vitamins and minerals) and

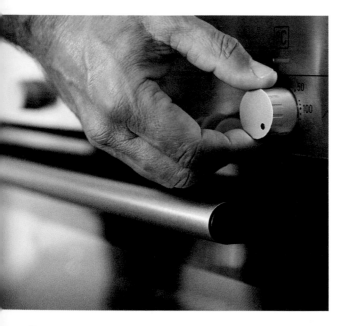

in extreme cases with draining "life force". The benefits, on the other hand, are said to be wide-ranging and include enhanced immune function, improved fertility, glowing skin and weight loss.

Meat and dairy are not allowed on raw-food diets, which are generally made up of at least 75% raw fruits, vegetables, germinated nuts and seeds and sprouts. Juicing and blending is allowed. Advocates of this diet suggest that any of the shortfalls in nutrient intake due to lack of protein or dairy (e.g. iron, calcium, fibre and some B vitamins) are offset by the intake of "superfoods" such as spinach, sesame seeds, goji berries, etc. However, as before, there is no evidence that not cooking your food has any additional health benefits over cooking it.

That said, fruits and vegetables are of course relatively low in calories, so relying on these for energy is likely to result in weight loss. It is also true that cooking does lead to the loss of some nutrients in our food; boiling green, leafy veg will result in the leaching of B vitamins, for instance. But it is not true to say that all forms of cooking are equal – if I stir-fry my broccoli the losses will be lower. Furthermore, cooking increases the bioavailability of some nutrients: more beta-carotene is absorbed from cooked carrots than from raw.

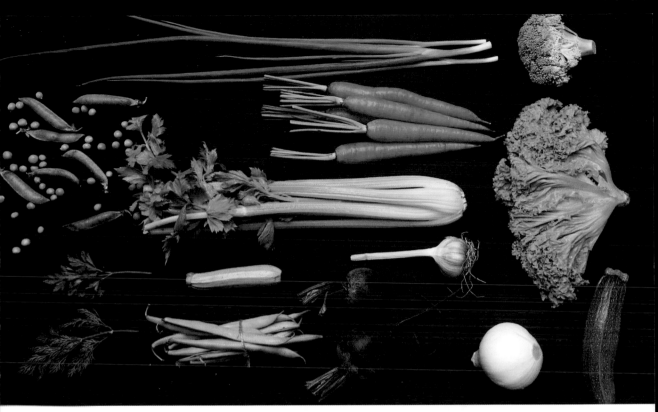

OPPOSITE: Some "back-to-nature" diet fads advise that foods should never be heated above 48°C (118°F).

ABOVE: The beta carotene in raw food is harder to absorb than in cooked.

RIGHT: Stir-frying is a popular method of light cooking, preserving levels of nutrients such as vitamin C.

The bottom line: Cooking our food allows for greater variety and diversity. It does not make it harder for the body to produce enzymes to digest our food – in some cases it makes food easier to digest. There is no scientific evidence that cooked food will substantially change the pH of body fluids and make the body more acidic. A balanced diet should contain a combination of cooked and raw food. Needless to say, as with most extreme diets, a raw-food diet is not suitable for children, who have high energy needs in order to support growth.

CAN YOU EAT YOURSELF HAPPY?

Food and mood are closely linked, but is there any evidence to indicate that single ingredients or micronutrients, or even whole food groups, will fix us in a state of happiness?

WHEN WE EAT a healthy, balanced diet, we tend to feel happier, but it is not known how much this is influenced by the nutrient content of our food and how much is purely psychological. Most people who lose weight through changing to a healthier lifestyle will have a feeling of happiness from their sense of achievement alone. Scientists are working on untangling the complex processes that control our emotions and investigating whether it is possible to separate the psychological from the biological elements at play. So what do we really know about the science behind food and mood?

MOOD FOOD

The effect of carbohydrate intake on mood has been extensively studied. The brain and nervous system are fuelled by the digestive system: incoming food is broken down and causes a rise in blood sugar, which our neurons use as energy, enabling us to concentrate and function. Insulin is produced in response to the rise in blood sugar, and it is this glucose–insulin relationship that is damaged in type 2 diabetes. We do know that refined carbohydrates with a high GI – for example white bread and many cereals – raise blood sugar dramatically for a short time, often referred to as a blood-sugar spike. When the blood sugar falls, some individuals report being left feeling irritable, anxious and hungry again. But, as with "good" foods and happiness, some of these feelings may stem from the guilt of eating a less healthy food.

Less-processed forms of carbohydrate, such as wholegrain bread and oats, raise blood sugar less sharply and for longer, which helps us to feel full and more satisfied, and could possibly encourage a calmer mood. Conversely, while carbohydrate foods such as pasta, mashed potato or sweets are called "comfort foods", it's because we reach for

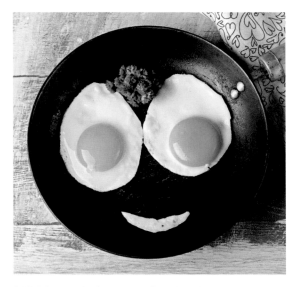

ABOVE: Does the food we eat actually make us happy or just make us feel happy with our choice?

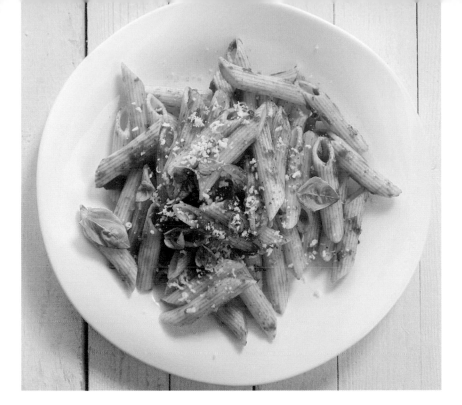

LEFT: A plate of pasta could boost the production of the happy hormone serotonin.

BELOW: Some foods such as pumpkin seeds are rich in tryptophan, needed for the production of serotonin.

them when we're tired or stressed; they can be a major energy source for our nervous system and stimulate the release of neurotransmitters, but the "comfort" effect is arguably just a result of treating ourselves or evoking memories from a time we felt happier, such as childhood.

THE HAPPY HORMONE

The food we eat can affect the chemical messaging in our bodies, which in turn affects our feelings and emotions. Carbohydrates, for example, promote the production of serotonin, the so-called happy hormone, which is a key ingredient in some depression medication, and it is therefore important not to cut carbs out completely. Single ingredients such as turkey and pumpkin seeds are often promoted as mood enhancers because they contain the amino acid tryptophan, which is a building block for serotonin production. Increasing the amount in our diet, therefore, seems logical. However, there is no evidence that incorporating higher amounts of tryptophan-containing foods actually raises our serotonin levels and makes us happier.

Serotonin is also produced in our intestines – researchers think as much as 95% of the body's supply is made there. Increasing the diversity of bacteria that live in our intestines by eating more probiotic foods, such as live yogurt, may have a positive effect on serotonin production. This is an exciting area of current research.

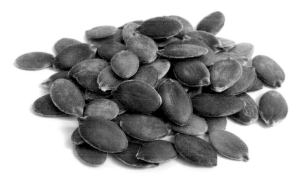

How serotonin is produced

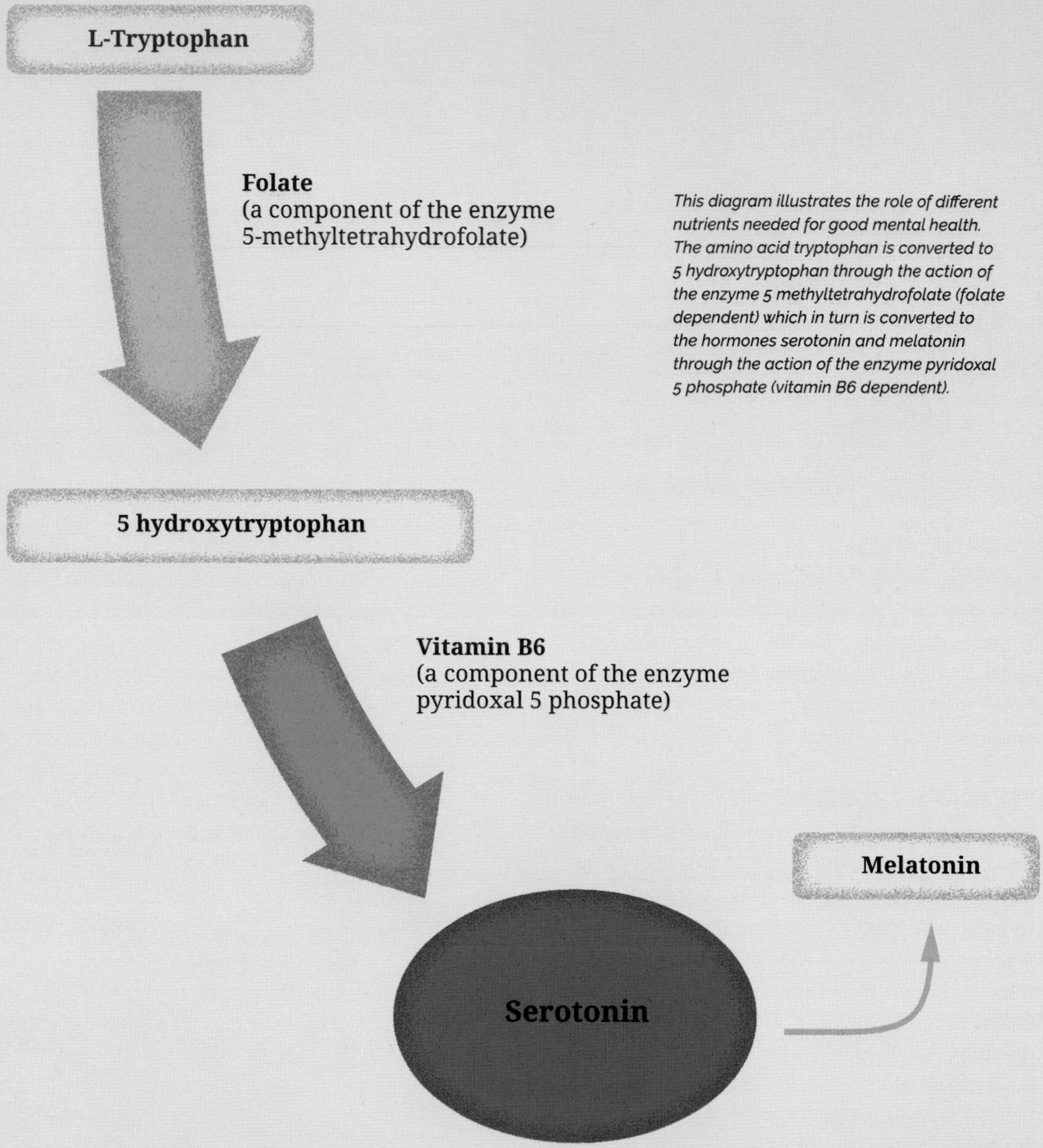

L-Tryptophan

Folate
(a component of the enzyme
5-methyltetrahydrofolate)

This diagram illustrates the role of different nutrients needed for good mental health. The amino acid tryptophan is converted to 5 hydroxytryptophan through the action of the enzyme 5 methyltetrahydrofolate (folate dependent) which in turn is converted to the hormones serotonin and melatonin through the action of the enzyme pyridoxal 5 phosphate (vitamin B6 dependent).

5 hydroxytryptophan

Vitamin B6
(a component of the enzyme
pyridoxal 5 phosphate)

Melatonin

Serotonin

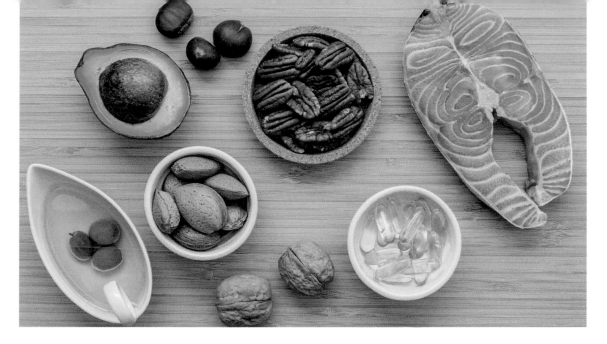

FOOD AND DEPRESSION

Something scientists have already determined is a link between obesity and depression, and they now recognize nutrition as a modifiable factor in lowering the risk of depression. An unhealthy diet leading to weight gain causes inflammation in the body, which exerts stress on the body's finely tuned pathways. The resulting production of inappropriate signals may affect the workings of the brain and its control of mood and behaviour. There is good evidence from studies of people's diets to suggest that individuals consuming a large amount of highly processed foods, such as takeaways and convenience meals, are more likely to have depression than individuals consuming a Mediterranean-style diet consisting of fruits, vegetables, lean meat, fish, olive oils and nuts. In terms of individual nutrients, there is some evidence that fish-eaters have a lower risk of depression, probably as a result of the omega-3 fatty acids they consume. Low levels of vitamin D and folate are also often found in individuals with depression. For vitamin D to be made in the skin, the skin must be exposed to high enough levels of UVB light from the sun – something that is notably absent in the northern latitudes during the winter months, when skin cannot make vitamin D even on a bright, sunny day. To date there is little evidence that supplementing our diet with any of these vitamins will alter risk, but it is likely that depression can be avoided in some individuals by mindful eating.

FIBRE FOR VITALITY

We are also learning more and more about the role of fibre in health and have good evidence for a decreased disease risk through raising the fibre content in our diet. It could be argued that the non-constipating effects of fibre can reduce tiredness and other sluggish symptoms and thereby increase a sense of wellbeing. In the most recent government guidelines for fibre, adults are advised to incorporate 30g (1oz) per day in their diets. The average intake of fibre is well below this amount, however, and as many as eight out of 10 of us do not meet the recommendation. Eating more fibre does not have to mean fancier ingredients – baked beans are a fantastic source of inexpensive fibre.

....

ABOVE: Foods such as salmon and walnuts are a good source of omega-3 fats.

CAN YOU DETOX YOUR BODY WITH JUICE?

Walk into any supermarket or open a popular magazine and you are likely to encounter products promising to "detox" your body – from companies who make them to celebrities who endorse them.

IN TODAY'S OBESOGENIC ENVIRONMENT, it is not surprising that individuals are drawn in to trying a new regime, and when so many people and products tell us that detoxing is good for us, we presume it must be so. Unfortunately, detox juices have no valid health claim. There is no quick and easy recipe for weight loss, and no scientific evidence to support the notion that fruit and vegetable juices actually increase detoxing, a process our bodies do ordinarily anyway.

WHAT IS DETOXING?

The term "detox" refers to the process of removing toxins (poisonous substances) that we do not want to build up in our bodies. The liver and kidneys are organs whose primary function is to do just that.

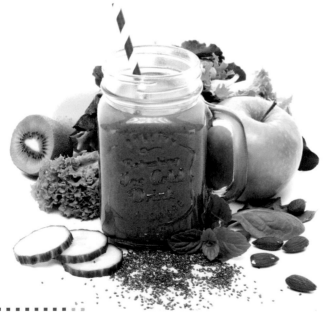

LEFT: A way to cleanse your system or just a healthy drink?

OPPOSITE ABOVE: The liver is the body's detoxifying organ.

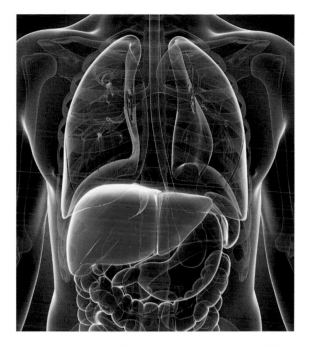

The liver recognizes and removes bacteria and other pathogens from the bloodstream and it also breaks down toxins. A good example is alcohol, whose poisonous component, acetaldehyde, is converted into carbon dioxide and water, which the body then gets rid of. The liver will keep pace with a moderate intake of alcohol, but in times of higher intake will struggle, and so some acetaldehyde will build up in the liver until it can be dealt with. A juicing detox following an over-indulgent social life will not confer any additional advantage over a few healthy-eating and alcohol-free days! The kidneys, meanwhile, filter unwanted substances out of the blood, regulate water balance and excrete waste in urine. There is no evidence that either the liver or kidneys require a rest or break from their functions.

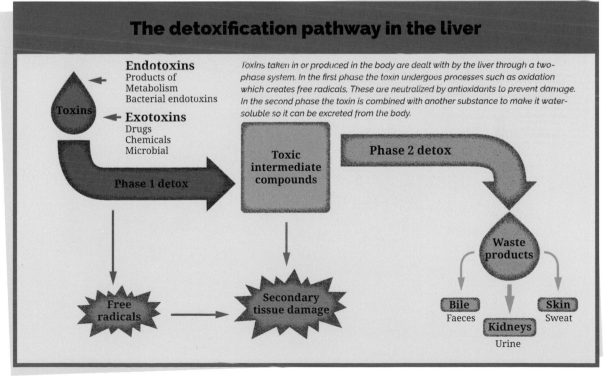

The detoxification pathway in the liver

Toxins

Endotoxins
Products of
Metabolism
Bacterial endotoxins

Exotoxins
Drugs
Chemicals
Microbial

Toxins taken in or produced in the body are dealt with by the liver through a two-phase system. In the first phase the toxin undergoes processes such as oxidation which creates free radicals, These are neutralized by antioxidants to prevent damage. In the second phase the toxin is combined with another substance to make it water-soluble so it can be excreted from the body.

Phase 1 detox

Toxic intermediate compounds

Phase 2 detox

Free radicals

Secondary tissue damage

Waste products

Bile
Faeces

Kidneys
Urine

Skin
Sweat

A JUICE DIET

Detoxing regimes can vary in length, from a few days to a week, with participants generally avoiding all solid foodstuffs and ingesting only liquid juices made from vegetables and fruit and usually taken several times a day. One of the main reasons why this is not considered a healthy choice is the lack of balance in nutritional intake – and the longer the period of time, the worse the situation becomes.

Juice is usually packed with vitamins and minerals, which are obviously good for our bodies, but the lack of protein, fat, fibre and complex carbohydrate is detrimental to the normal functioning of the body. This can result in individuals feeling tired, dizzy and nauseous. In addition, some essential nutrients require help from other nutrients to be fully beneficial; for example, vitamins A, D, E and K are called the fat-soluble vitamins, and without fat their absorption will be limited. Juices vary in

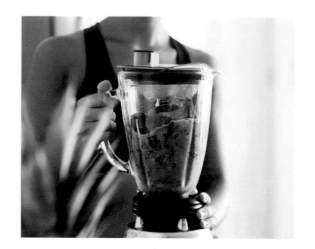

nutritional value but those containing a lot of fruit will also contain a lot of sugar. Sugar in liquid form, when it is not attached to any fibrous component such as fruit skin, is absorbed readily by the body,

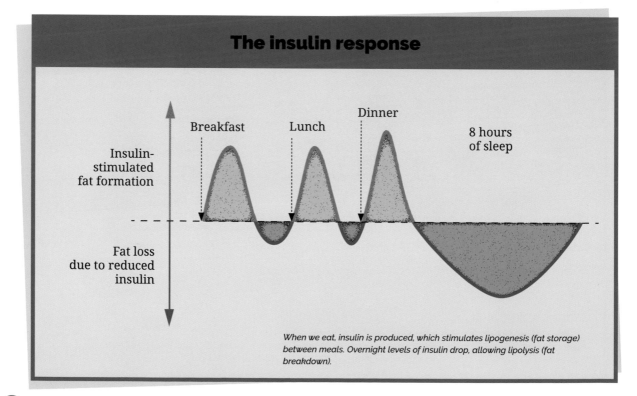

The insulin response

Breakfast

Lunch

Dinner

8 hours of sleep

Insulin-stimulated fat formation

Fat loss due to reduced insulin

When we eat, insulin is produced, which stimulates lipogenesis (fat storage) between meals. Overnight levels of insulin drop, allowing lipolysis (fat breakdown).

causing a blood-sugar spike. The consequent insulin response can leave some individuals feeling moody and hungry.

JUICES AND WEIGHT LOSS

Detoxing juices will likely constitute a very low-calorie daily intake, so even a few days' worth of such a diet will result in rapid weight loss. Endorsers of detox juices often highlight this accompanying weight loss as an attraction of the regime, but most people do end up putting the weight back on when they return to a normal diet. There is no evidence of long-term weight management. Plus the weight loss isn't as attractive as it sounds. Our bodies first make available energy from ingested food, then glycogen stores. Next, muscle mass will be broken down in order to keep us functioning and the metabolism will actually slow to conserve energy. So much of the initial weight loss from radical juice diets is water weight. This is because glycogen is stored in water, and as glycogen levels deplete, the water in which it was held is lost. There is also a reduction in muscle mass. In addition, individuals may be left feeling weak, with little or no energy, and may experience headaches as a result of their overall very low calorie intake. These symptoms are not a result of toxin expulsion, as is commonly reported.

Arguably, one benefit to a short-term juice detox may be that individuals have the chance to break a cycle of unhealthy eating, and when returning to a normal calorie intake there is some evidence that they are more mindful about their choices and feel satiated with less food than usual. This post-detox perk can provide a motivational boost to proceed with a new healthful future.

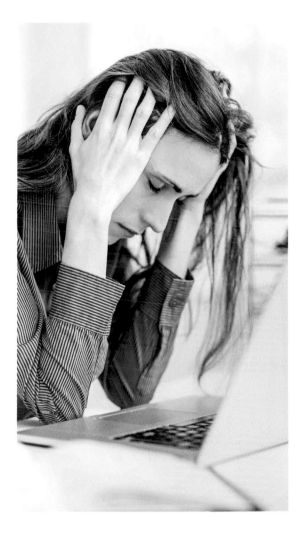

OPPOSITE ABOVE: Juicing is a popular choice for detoxing, with "juice cleansing" one of today's biggest wellness trends.

ABOVE: Juice lacks key nutrients, without which you may be left feeling fatigued.

The bottom line: The liver and kidneys are the body's organs responsible for dealing with excreting toxins. As long as they stay healthy, they will work normally every day without the need for "detox" juice. While there is no real harm in having a couple of juice days as a kickstart for a new period of healthy eating, be aware that you might not feel great, so pick a quiet weekend on which to do it.

DO WE ALL NEED SUPPLEMENTS?

Most high streets have at least one health-food shop stocked with shelves of supplements; supermarkets have at least one shelf and pharmacies usually a dedicated section. Supplements are big business. So do we all need them?

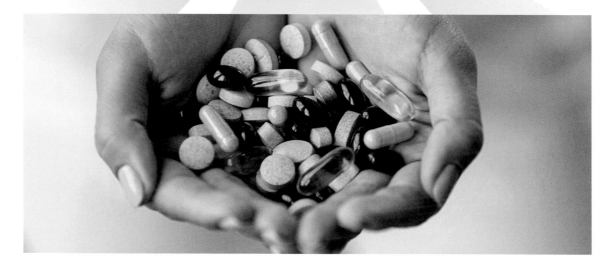

AT FIRST GLANCE, the sheer range of supplements may suggest that we do – after all, there are supplements tailored for gender, age, life stage and health condition, for sports, or boasting specific ingredients ranging from echinacea to prebiotics.

WHO MIGHT BENEFIT?

Supplements can play a role in helping to keep us healthy, particularly at times when following a healthy, balanced diet is difficult, or when people are restricting their dietary intake or have suffered nutrient losses. For example, some vegetarians may benefit from an iron supplement, while individuals with poor bone mass or osteopenia (decreased bone density) may

benefit from vitamin D and calcium supplements. Furthermore, there are life stages during which a supplement is key, such as folic acid before and during the early stages of pregnancy to avoid neural tube defects in the growing foetus, or vitamin D drops in infants and young children to avoid rickets (a skeletal disorder). But assuming we eat a variety of foods, most of us do not need supplements.

What about sports nutrition supplements? Protein, specifically in the form of whey supplements, is a multi-billion-dollar business, but this waste product of cheese production is not an essential supplement for muscle recovery and synthesis – protein from food will do exactly the same job.

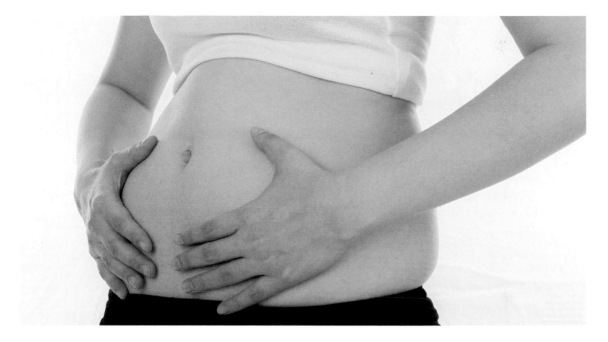

NUTRITION IN A PILL?

One may also question whether the benefits often attributed to supplements really exist. Although some claims sound rather spurious, particularly those on supplements bought on the internet, others make health claims with a more solidly scientific foundation. For example, a claim approved in Europe is the benefit of taking 2g/day (0.7oz) of fish-oil supplements to help maintain normal blood-triglyceride levels. In Europe, a series of laws exist dictating that any health claims attributed to supplements must be approved by regulators – they should be based on science and must not mislead. Furthermore, supplements should not be harmful or contaminated with other ingredients, and they should not encourage deviation from a healthy, balanced diet.

OPPOSITE: Supplements range from individual nutrients such as vitamin C to multivitamins and minerals or a combination of nutrients needed for aspects of health such as calcium and vitamin D for bone health.

ABOVE: Supplements are officially recommended for certain groups of people, for instance folic acid for the first 12 weeks of pregnancy.

RIGHT: Whey protein is a means of supplementing branched-chain amino acids.

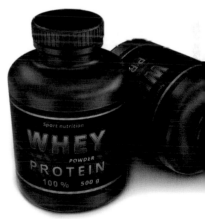

The bottom line: Supplements can be helpful in fulfilling a specific role, but there is usually no need for their long-term use unless under medical supervision. Those with wide-ranging or extreme claims should be viewed with caution – if it sounds too good to be true, then unfortunately that is most likely to be the case!

IS FASTING GOOD FOR YOU?

The phrase "I'm on a fast day" has become a socially acceptable means of refusing food or turning down an invitation to eat. Fasting has become a very popular method of controlling what you eat and can be an effective way to lose weight, but is what we call fasting really fasting or just another variant of a very low-calorie diet?

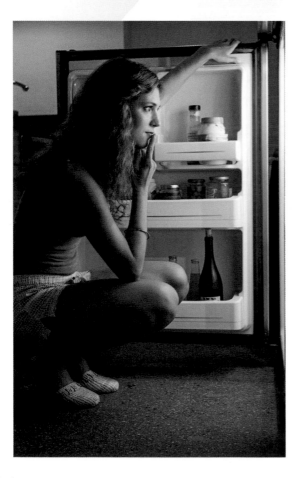

FASTING: THE FACTS

The distinction between fasting and starvation is that the former usually entails the willing abstinence from all food and drink for a defined period only. Fasting is a practice in certain religions and is also recommended by doctors for a patient requiring a blood test or imminent surgery. The Islamic festival of Ramadan, when many millions of Muslims fast for a month during daylight hours, has provided an opportunity for research into the effects of fasting on health and wellbeing. Studies have been carried out on various groups, including normal healthy adults as well as potentially more vulnerable groups such as pregnant women and the elderly (although it should be pointed out that there is no obligation on these groups to fast). The majority of these studies have reported significant metabolic changes, including dehydration and raised levels of uric acid and cholesterol in the blood. While these have not translated into short- or long-term health problems, neither could they be considered health benefits. The most commonly reported fasting-related complaints are of irritability, headaches, lack of concentration, fatigue and poor sleep.

As the popularity of intermittent fasting has grown, various fasting regimens have been devised,

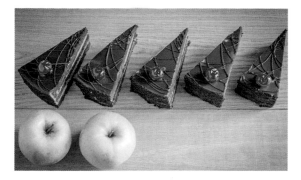

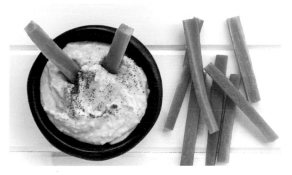

including alternate-day fasting, the 5:2 diet (fasting for two days of the week) and the 16:8 diet (fasting for 16 hours of the day). By far the best known is the 5:2, whose popularity stems from the fact that it is easy to comply with. Unlike more traditional calorie-restricted regimes under which you have to adhere to the same restriction every day, the 5:2 allows you to eat normally for five days a week, with restricted calories on the other two days. So even the fast days are not really fasts: you are allowed to consume 20–25% of your energy requirement (which translates to 500 calories for women and 600 calories for men). How you consume these calories is up to you; most people tend to split their calories between two meals, for instance a late breakfast/brunch and an early supper.

When following one of these severely calorie-restricted fast-day diets, it is recommended that on fast days you choose foods that help you feel fuller for longer. These are foods that help satiation (the more immediate feeling of fullness that stops you eating more at the same meal) and satiety

OPPOSITE: Fasting requires steely determination and resolve not to give in to hunger pangs; an appropriately stocked fridge can help.

ABOVE LEFT: The 5:2 approach involves semi-fasting for two days of the week and eating normally for the other five.

ABOVE RIGHT: Hummus is a good source of protein and fibre, and will help you feel fuller more quickly.

(the longer-lasting feeling of fullness that stops you eating again soon afterwards). Foods that improve satiation include high-protein, high-liquid foods such as yogurts, hummus, scrambled eggs, vegetable soups and stews. Foods that improve satiety include low-sugar, high-fibre foods such as pulses, nuts, vegetables and wholegrains.

Initially the fasting days are challenging, as even with the food allowed you will experience hunger pangs, but after a few weeks this can pass. Some people have reported feeling quite empowered by fasting, while others even have a sense of freedom and relief from the dilemma of choosing what to eat.

The bottom line: A small number of scientific studies on the various forms of intermittent fasting have shown positive results for weight loss and other health outcomes, including improved cholesterol levels and possible reduced risk of diabetes. But these effects are as a result of the body being allowed to enter and remain in a "fasted" state for a significant period of time. Being in a fasted (as opposed to a well-fed) state causes different hormones to be released and it is this shift in hormonal balance that benefits health. Our current culture of snacking and grazing between meals, even on foods we consider healthy, disrupts the fasted state.

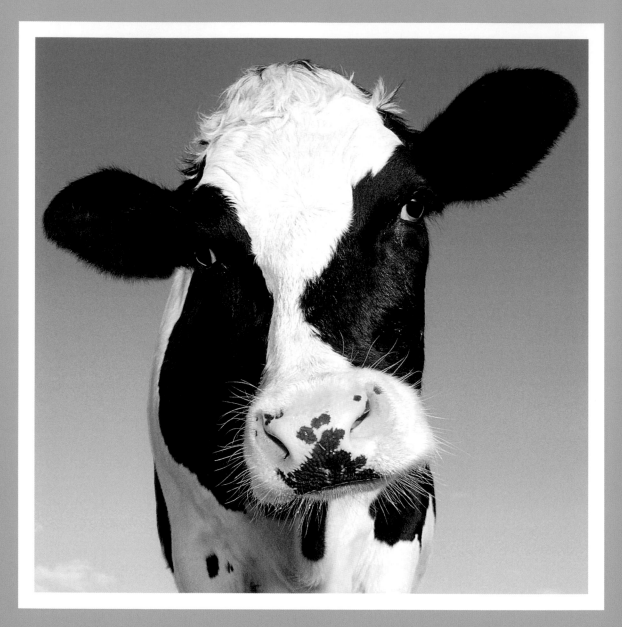

11

CUT
IT OUT

Myths relating to meat and dairy

ARE WE NOT DESIGNED TO EAT MEAT?

There is no doubt that powerful arguments exist for stopping, or greatly reducing, our consumption of meat. Animal farming has an incredibly destructive effect on the environment and excessive meat consumption is strongly linked with bowel cancer.

THE WORLD CANCER RESEARCH FUND recommends that we eat no more than 500g (18oz) a week of red meat, which includes beef, pork and lamb, and avoid processed meat, such as ham and bacon, altogether. However, a less convincing argument is that man is not designed to eat meat. Over millions of years, we have evolved from primate to modern-day man on a journey that is widely documented in the form of fossils, burial sites, prehistoric faeces, tools, firepits and ancient rubbish dumps. Fossil records from the African continent indicate that the change from primate to bipedal hominid occurred around six million years ago, and that today's anatomically modern human emerged 200,000 years ago. What was the trigger for this change in our evolution? The most likely answer is a change in diet – and specifically a change in the type of protein consumed.

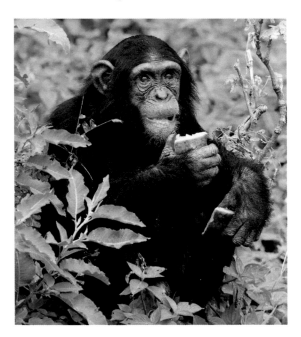

WHEN DID WE START TO EAT MEAT?

The predominantly herbivore diet of early primates would have been foraged from forests and consisted of fruit, seeds, tree bark, plant bulbs, shoots and flowers. It may have been

LEFT: The shift from herbivorous to omnivorous diet may have helped our evolution to modern man.

OPPOSITE LEFT: Foraging for fruit would not have provided enough energy for early man.

OPPOSITE RIGHT: Meat and fish provided a major source of energy for hunter-gatherer man.

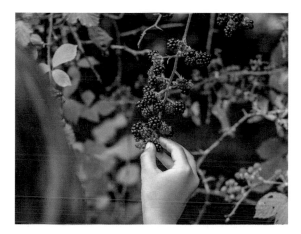

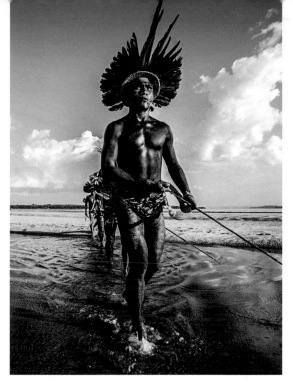

supplemented with insects. Studies of the pre-human diet show that meat was being consumed two million years ago and as humans developed this consumption steadily increased. As we evolved, our genetic make-up adapted to improve our survival rates and one such adaptation was our physiological ability to eat meat. This evolutionary sequence was probably triggered by a change in diet that significantly boosted the availability of high-quality protein. The increased consumption of protein (and specifically high-quality protein) that would have provided good amounts of the essential amino acids led to enhanced brain growth, which enabled a rapid acquisition of skills, such as tool-making, language and cultural expression. As man developed into a hunter-gatherer, the consumption of meat contributed a major source of energy, which meant that there was more time to spend on social interaction, which in turn stimulated brain growth and the acquisition of skills.

Lean red meat would also have contributed to improved nutritional status, specifically providing significant amounts of nutrients needed to support heart health and the immune system, including essential omega-3 fatty acids, iron, zinc, selenium, thiamine, vitamin B12 and vitamin D.

A review of dietary studies on hunter-gatherers suggests that food from animals provided two thirds of daily energy intakes, with the rest comprised of gathered plant sources. This is supported by evidence from from the analyses of different markers in the body such as the activity of certain enzymes that would have been needed to digest the food. Intakes of protein are estimated to have provided 19–35% of energy, while carbohydrates provided an average of 30%. In modern diets, carbohydrates provide closer to 50% of energy.

The bottom line: The decision whether or not to eat meat is entirely personal, based on a number of factors including beliefs, ethics and taste. It is perfectly possible to maintain good health with or without the inclusion of meat; however, there is no doubt that the introduction of meat in the diet of our ancient ancestors hugely benefited our evolution into modern man.

ARE VEGANS HEALTHIER?

Veganism was once thought to be a fad confined to animal-loving, flower-wearing hippies living in communes. But now it has had a surge in popularity, with A-list celebrities jumping on the bandwagon and transforming veganism from weird-cult status to destination lifestyle. But before you consider eliminating all animal products from your life, there are things you need to know.

WHAT IS VEGANISM?

The UK Vegan Society defines veganism as "a philosophy and way of living which seeks to exclude – as far as possible and practicable – all forms of exploitation of, and cruelty to, animals for food, clothing or any other purpose; and by extension, promotes the development and use of animal-free alternatives for the benefit of humans, animals and the environment. In dietary terms it denotes the practice of dispensing with all products derived wholly or partly from animals." So veganism is a plant-based diet that avoids all animal-derived foods such as meat (including fish, shellfish and insects), dairy, eggs and honey.

However, being vegan does not just mean eating vegetables. The diet should also include lots of other plant-based foods such as tofu, rice, quinoa, nuts and seeds.

VEGANISM: THE TRUTH

Being nutritionally healthy means both meeting your daily requirement for all the essential nutrients your body needs and having a good intake of substances in the diet that, although not classified as essential, nonetheless confer health benefits. These substances include phytochemicals (compounds found in plants),

such as flavonoids, which have antioxidant and anti-inflammatory properties. With careful planning and understanding of what makes up a healthy, balanced vegan diet, you can get all the nutrients your body needs. A vegan diet is much likelier than a non-vegan one to be higher in phytochemicals and some nutrients, such as fibre.

However, contrary to popular belief, it's still very easy to eat unhealthily on a vegan diet. Vegans may argue that veganism is a way of life, not a diet you can dip in and out of. This means that, without real

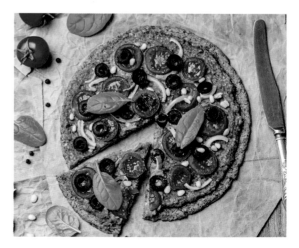

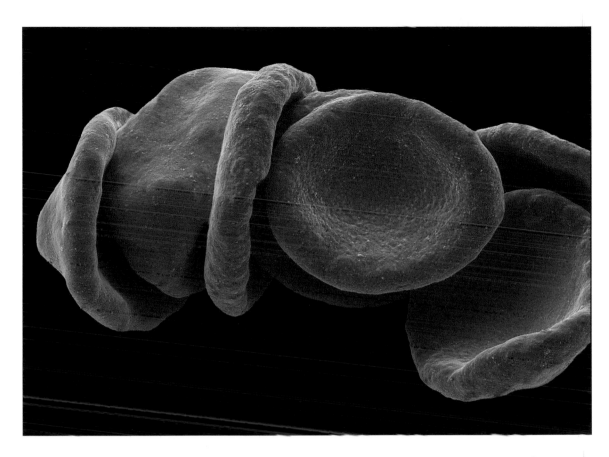

effort to plan and prepare each meal, especially those eaten outside the home, it is easy to resort to lazy choices such as a packet of crisps or a fizzy drink. Vegans are advised to take supplements, and some may easily become deficient in a few important nutrients due to restrictions on what they eat. Plant-based foods contain smaller quantities of some nutrients and are less easily absorbed than those from animal products. Iron and calcium are the most concerning mineral losses, together with vitamin B12.

IRON

Iron is an integral part of haemoglobin, which is needed in red blood cells for transporting oxygen around the body. It is also necessary for growth, development, normal cellular functioning and the synthesis of some hormones and connective tissue. A low intake can lead to tiredness and fatigue or even anaemia. Women of childbearing age have a higher dietary requirement for iron than men, due to monthly losses of blood through menstruation. With intakes of iron already low in 46% of teenage girls and 23% of women in the UK, females in particular need to take care when embarking on a vegan diet as they may be at higher risk of iron-deficiency anaemia.

....

OPPOSITE: A vegan pizza may be delicious, but vegan diets are not automatically healthy. As with meat-containing diets, it all depends on an adequate supply of nutrients.

ABOVE: Vegan diets may lack iron and vitamin B12, both of which are needed for production of red blood cells such as these.

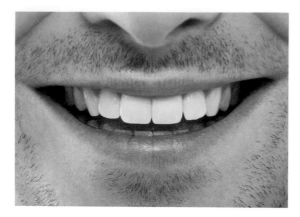

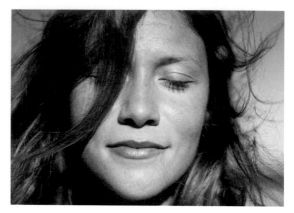

Dietary iron has two main forms: haem and non-haem. Haem iron is found in meat, poultry and seafood and is easily absorbed during digestion because the iron exists in the form of ferrous iron (Fe^{2+}). Non-haem iron is found in plant foods and foods fortified with iron such as breakfast cereals. Non-haem iron is not readily absorbed as it exists in the form of ferric iron (Fe^{3+}) and must be reduced to ferrous iron before it can taken up by the intestinal cells. The presence of vitamin C can reduce ferric iron to ferrous iron and so aid absorption. Studies have shown that when a mixed diet is consumed that includes meat and other animal foods, about 14–18% of iron is absorbed; however, only around 5% of the iron in a vegan diet is absorbed. And unlike with haem iron, some substances present in plant-based foods, such as grains and beans, can hinder the absorption of non-haem iron. On paper, spinach looks like a good source of iron, but in fact it has low iron bioavailability (ease of absorption). Tea and coffee can also contain polyphenols, which inhibit iron absorption, so it is best to avoid drinking tea and coffee with meals.

CALCIUM

Calcium is essential for maintaining strong and healthy bones and teeth, and so is especially important for teenagers who are still developing. Bones are not fully formed until your early twenties, when bone density is at its highest.

People consuming mixed diets obtain most of their calcium through the consumption of dairy products, as the bioavailability of calcium from foods like milk, cheese and dairy is good. Calcium is present in plant foods such as green leafy veg, nuts and seeds, but its bioavailability varies widely. The best source of calcium for vegans is foods in which extra calcium has been added, such as fortified plant milks (nut, soya, oat and rice), and foods made with fortified flour.

VITAMIN D

Although most vitamin D is obtained through the action of sunlight on the skin, this can only occur during the summer months at northern latitudes. There are few natural food sources of vitamin D, the richest being oily fish and meat. Vegans can obtain vitamin D in their diet from fortified foods such as margarines, breakfast cereals and soya drinks. Vitamin D can also be obtained from mushrooms that have been specially exposed to ultraviolet light to boost their content. It is probably wise to consider taking a supplement.

ABOVE LEFT: Calcium is not only important for strong bones, it is also needed for healthy teeth such as these.

ABOVE RIGHT: Vitamin D is made in the body on exposure to sunlight during the summer months; during the winter, even in sunny weather, we have to rely on dietary intake.

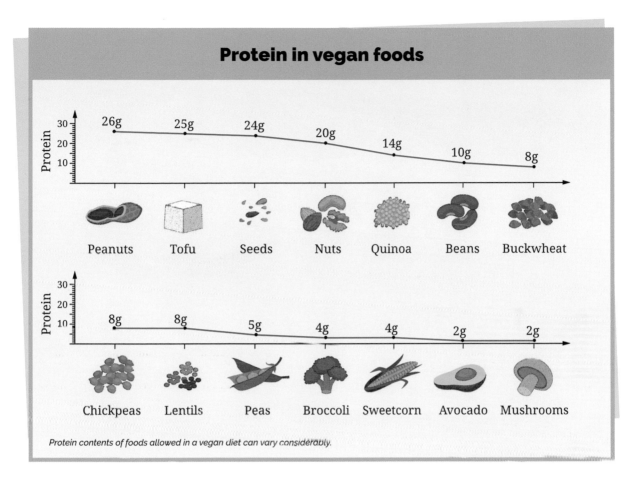

Protein in vegan foods

Peanuts — 26g
Tofu — 25g
Seeds — 24g
Nuts — 20g
Quinoa — 14g
Beans — 10g
Buckwheat — 8g

Chickpeas — 8g
Lentils — 8g
Peas — 5g
Broccoli — 4g
Sweetcorn — 4g
Avocado — 2g
Mushrooms — 2g

Protein contents of foods allowed in a vegan diet can vary considerably.

VITAMIN B12

Vitamin B12 is the only vitamin where it is routinely recommended that a supplement is taken. This is because it is only found naturally in animal foods. A few vegan-friendly foods have vitamin B12 added, including breakfast cereals, plant milks and yeast-extract spreads like Marmite or Vegemite.

PROTEIN

Going vegan could impact intake of good-quality protein. Animal products contain all of the essential amino acids (i.e. those that the body cannot make itself), which are the building blocks of protein in the body. Most plant-based foods contain a small amount of one or two of the essential amino acids needed by the body. You can still optimize your protein intake on a vegan diet, but you should ensure you are consuming a wide range of protein-based foods.

Soya and quinoa contain all the essential amino acids and are known as complete sources of protein. However, many other vegan sources of protein do not, and therefore it is important to combine different types of protein foods as part of the same meal (known as protein complementation) in order to get enough of all the essential amino acids. It is also important not to rely on just one type of protein to avoid missing out on essential nutrients.

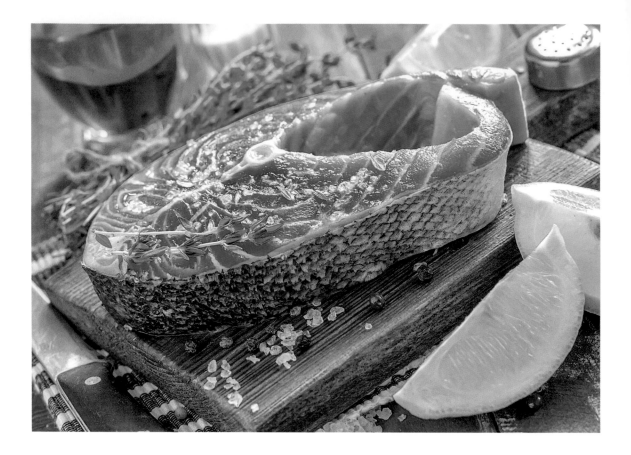

OMEGA-3 FATTY ACIDS

It is recommended that we eat at least one portion of oily fish per week in order to obtain an adequate amount of the long-chain omega-3 polyunsaturated fatty acids found in these fish. These fats are important for maintaining a healthy heart and help to reduce the risk of heart disease when consumed as part of a healthy diet.

Vegan sources of omega-3 fatty acids include various plant oils, such as flaxseed, rapeseed and

ABOVE: The exclusion of oily fish can make if difficult to get adequate intakes of omega-3 fats.

soya, as well as walnuts. However, there is evidence to suggest that plant sources of omega-3 fatty acids may not have the same heart-health benefits as those found in oily fish because they cannot easily be converted into the type found in oily fish.

The bottom line: Despite the opportunity it offers to eat more fruit, veg and wholegrains, a vegan diet is not necessarily healthier – and it means careful planning to ensure that it provides enough of the nutrients needed to meet the body's requirements.

IS DAIRY BAD FOR YOU?

In 2016 I made some comments on a TV programme in defence of milk. The social-media backlash that followed was a shock, with a group of staunchly committed vegans posting increasingly offensive and abusive comments. While I can understand ethical and environmental concerns around dairy farming, all credibility is lost when ludicrous claims are made about the nutrition of dairy. Whether you like it or loathe it, milk and dairy products are far from bad for you, and their consumption is not associated with any of the following conditions.

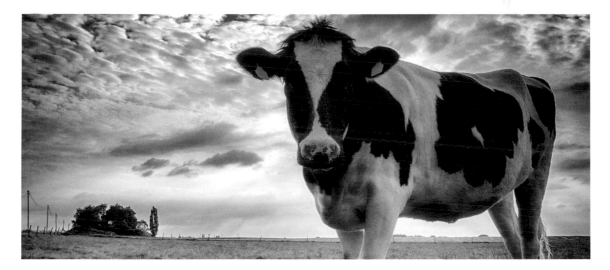

ACNE

Acne is a skin condition characterized by red inflamed spots during puberty. It is believed to be caused by the hormone testosterone. Testosterone signals to glands in the skin to produce oil, but if too much is produced skin pores can become blocked, causing spots, blackheads or blister-like lesions to form. Some people believe that consumption of milk and dairy contributes to the development and severity of spots, although no convincing evidence exists to support this myth. Most experts believe that diet has little impact on acne and that other factors such as genetics, skin type, hormone levels and exposure to environmental pollutants are more likely to be involved. Therefore, excluding milk and dairy foods is not advisable in the treatment of acne as this may compromise intake of essential nutrients.

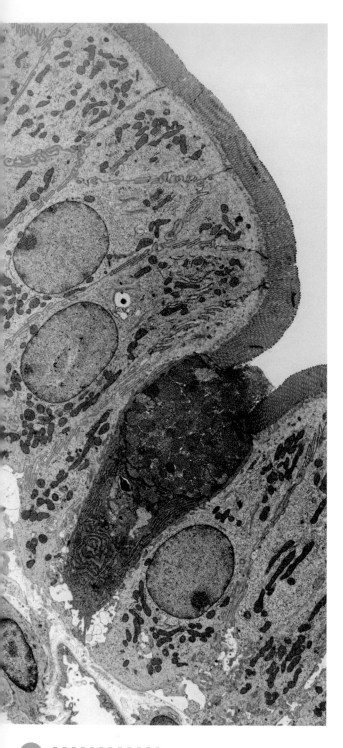

EXCESS MUCUS

Mucus is a fluid secreted by the mucous membranes in the body and it covers the surface of the respiratory and digestive systems to provide protection against damage, infection and irritation. There is a common myth, apparently dating back to the twelfth century, that milk and dairy products increase the production of mucus in the respiratory system and should therefore be removed from the diet. Traditional Chinese medical beliefs also deem these foods to increase mucus production, together with chocolate, honey and other natural sweeteners. This myth has no scientific basis, as studies have failed to demonstrate any effect, but it is worrying nonetheless as it may lead to the unnecessary exclusion of a whole food group. That said, milk may thicken saliva, which can coat the throat and give the perception of more mucus, but it does not cause the body to produce more mucus or phlegm.

ECZEMA

There are many types of eczema, the most common of which is atopic eczema (or atopic dermatitis). This is a condition that causes the skin to become itchy, red, dry and cracked. The exact cause is unknown but it is thought to be genetic – i.e. it runs in families – and it can develop alongside other conditions such as asthma or hay fever. According to research conducted by the Nutrition and Health Department in Switzerland, atopic eczema affects 15–20% of children and 1–3% of adults worldwide. The symptoms are triggered by a number of factors, such as irritants (for example soaps, detergents and shampoos), environmental factors (cold and dry weather, dampness, house dust mites, pet fur, pollen and moulds), food allergies (such as allergy to cow's milk, eggs, peanuts, soya or wheat), hormonal changes, skin infections and emotional stress. There is currently no cure for atopic eczema but treatment can help relieve the symptoms and many children find their symptoms improve as they get older. However, you should not make significant changes to your diet without first

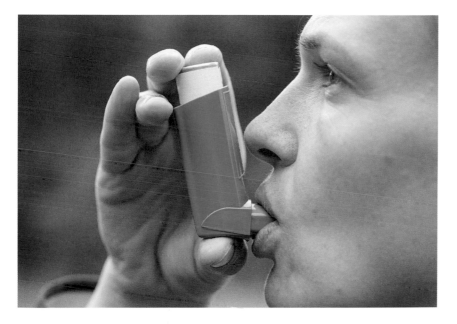

OPPOSITE: A goblet cell (yellow) secretes mucus, which protects the lining of the intestine and helps neutralize stomach acid.

LEFT: There is no evidence that milk causes or worsens asthma.

BELOW: Eczema can be a symptom of an allergy to milk, but milk is not the only possible cause.

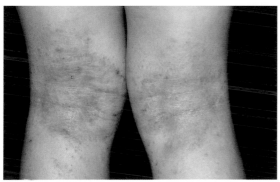

speaking to your doctor. If they suspect you have a food allergy you may be referred to see a dietician, who can help work out a balanced diet plan that avoids specific food. You may also be referred to see an immunologist, dermatologist or paediatrician.

ASTHMA

Asthma is a condition affecting the respiratory system and is characterized by swelling of the airways and excess mucus production. There can be a family history of asthma or it can be triggered by environmental factors such as allergens, e.g. dust.

For years it has been suggested that milk causes asthma or worsens the symptoms, but there is no scientific evidence to support this. However, those with a cow's-milk-protein allergy may have asthma-like symptoms. You should always ensure you are tested for allergies before excluding whole food groups such as dairy from your diet.

EXCESS HORMONES

The myth that milk contains harmful hormones seems to stem from the use of bovine somatotropin (BST), a growth hormone employed by some dairy farmers to boost milk production. This practice, which is forbidden in the EU, should in any case not have any impact on human health since BST is species-specific. In the USA, considerable testing was done in the early 1990s, comparing milk from BST-treated cows with that of untreated cows, and in 1993 the FDA (Food and Drug Administration) approved its use. Since then, other organizations including the World Health Organization, the Food and Agriculture Organization of the United Nations and the American Medical Association have all supported this FDA position.

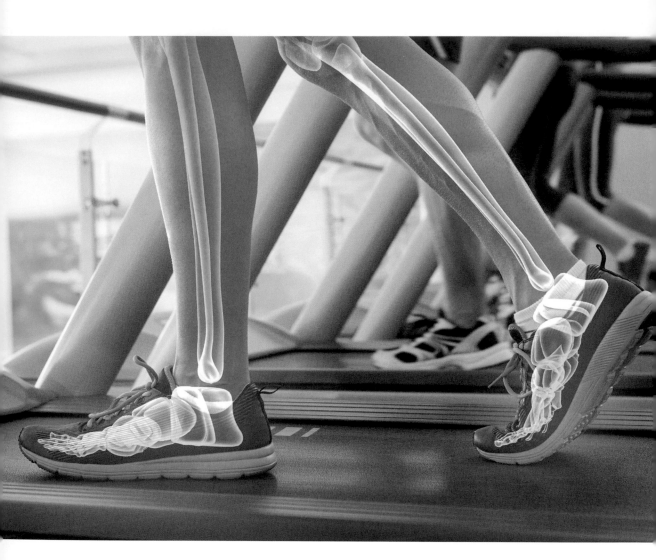

EARLY PUBERTY

Girls are now known to be entering puberty at a younger age than they did a generation ago. There are many hypotheses as to why this is, including childhood obesity, since puberty seems to happen earlier in heavier girls. Another hypothesis suggests that BST in milk is the culprit. However, there is no evidence to support this theory. In fact, children who consume more milk tend to have lower rather than higher body weight. So if obesity plays a role in early puberty, it is unlikely that milk contributes to this.

INGESTION OF ANTIBIOTICS

Cows, like humans, become unwell, and antibiotics can help combat bacterial infection and bring them back to full health. As you would expect, the use of veterinary medicines for animals used for food is tightly controlled by law. The milk of cows that have been given antibiotics is not allowed back into the food chain for a designated period, so as to avoid any carry-over of these antibiotics into milk for human consumption.

ACID/ALKALINE DIET

Another weight-loss craze backed by numerous celebrities is the acid/alkaline diet (see pages 14–17). This is based on the notion that eating certain foods, including meat and dairy, can increase the body's acidity levels, thereby increasing the risk of cancer and osteoporosis. Advocates recommend cutting out "acidic" foods such as meat, dairy and sugar, and following a strict regime of foods such as vegetables, fruit, beans and pulses. In fact, the body is clever at keeping blood pH within the extremely narrow range of 7.35–7.45, which is slightly alkaline. While nutritionists agree that certain foods do produce acid or alkali when they are digested, as always it's about consuming a balanced diet rather than cutting out entire food groups, which could lead to deficiency in many essential nutrients.

OPPOSITE: Milk and dairy products are key sources of both protein and calcium, which are needed for strong bones.

BELOW: Dairy products are a valuable source of many nutrients needed for good health, so think carefully before cutting dairy out of your diet.

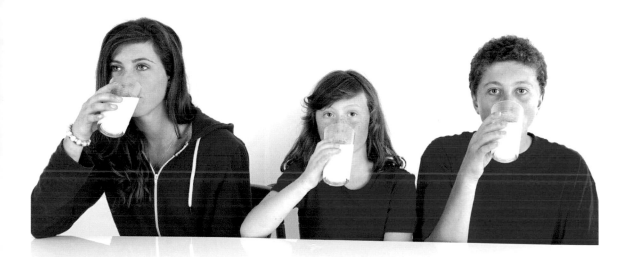

The bottom line: Milk and dairy products provide a range of essential nutrients important for good health, including calcium for the development and maintenance of healthy bones, protein for growth and repair, iodine to make thyroid hormones for healthy metabolism and vitamin B12 for healthy blood cells and nerve function. Milk ticks all the boxes for healthy snacking, providing hydration, vitamins and minerals (somewhat lacking in many other popular snacks) and protein. The protein will keep you feeing satisfied and fuller for longer, which is just what a snack should do. Milk can match pretty much any of the meal-replacement shakes and post-workout drinks available and does it naturally – nothing added, nothing modified. It provides protein for repairing muscles, fluid and electrolytes for rehydration, and natural sugar for replenishing energy levels.

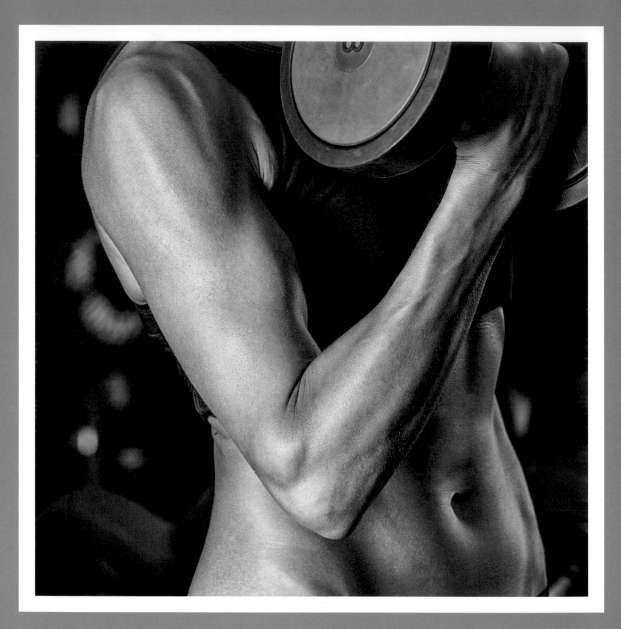

12

WORK IT OUT

Myths relating to exercise

EXERCISE: AN OVERVIEW

The concept of intentional exercise has grown steadily in popularity over the last 40–50 years. In the first half of the twentieth century, sports were only really practised by schoolboys and professional athletes. For the vast majority of human history, we only expended large amounts of energy in activities centred on our own survival and comfort – such as maintaining a shelter and procuring food and water – but advances in agriculture, industry and technology in recent centuries have led to the majority of the world's population now having sedentary rather than active lifestyles.

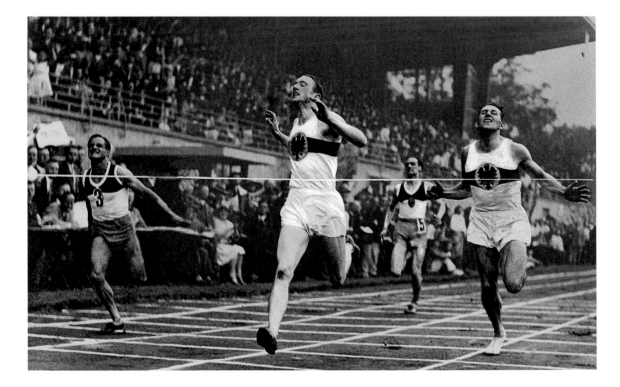

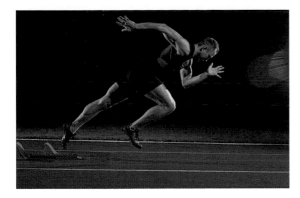

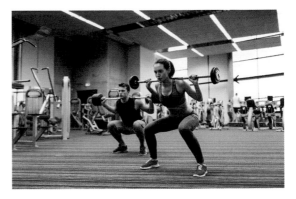

FAR FEWER PEOPLE TODAY have a job, for instance, that involves physical labour, and the use of cars and computers has become the norm. For most people who wish to expend energy, exercise is the only solution, be it a leisurely walk or training for a triathlon. As people become less and less active in their day-to-day lives, it is crucial that they find ways of exercising, particularly as inactivity is strongly associated with increased chronic-disease risk and disorders such as metabolic syndrome, non-alcoholic fatty liver disease and type 2 diabetes.

Currently it is recommended that we undertake around 150 minutes of moderate-to-vigorous aerobic exercise per week, spread across the days, in addition to resistance training on at least two days.

HOW DO WE FUEL OUR EXERCISE?

During exercise, various energy systems operate within the working muscle, depending on the type and intensity of the exercise being performed. These energy systems can be aerobic processes, which need oxygen, or anaerobic processes, which do not. For "explosive exercise" that only lasts a few seconds but requires energy faster than our bodies can provide it using oxygen, such as lifting a heavy weight or performing a power jump, the (anaerobic) phosphagen system is used to provide energy. This system relies on the amount of creatine phosphate stored in the muscle and cannot be sustained over time: there is generally only enough to sustain activity for a few seconds.

Another anaerobic pathway comes into use during high-intensity exercise. This system uses glycogen that is stored in the muscle and glucose provided by the blood. They are rapidly broken down but the process by which they are metabolized means that large amounts of lactic acid can build up, hindering the work rate of the muscle. For this reason, the working muscle cells can only continue this type of anaerobic energy production at high rates for 1–3 minutes. Approximately 25% of total muscle glycogen stores are used during a single 30-second sprint or resistance-exercise bout. Neither of these anaerobic pathways can sustain the rapid provision of energy to allow muscles to contract at a very high rate for more than 2–3 minutes.

The build-up of lactic acid during high-intensity exercise may seem counterproductive: why would a working muscle produce something that slows its capacity for more work? It is likely that this is actually a clever way of preventing permanent damage during extreme exertion by slowing the key systems needed to maintain muscle contraction.

....

OPPOSITE: Research into sports nutrition has grown rapidly over the last few decades, and as a result international athletics has changed enormously since the mid-twentieth century.

ABOVE: Explosive exercise such as sprinting and weight lifting relies on different energy systems than those needed for endurance exercise.

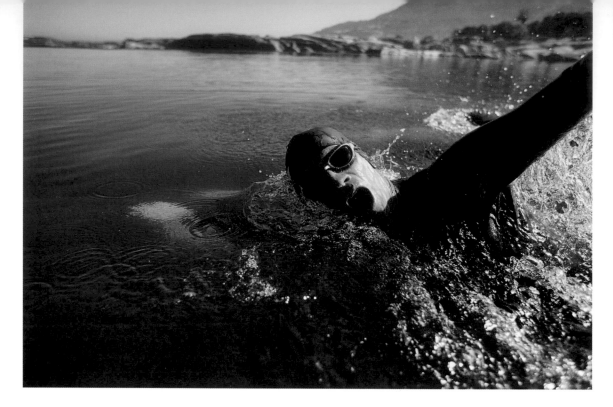

Once the body slows down, oxygen becomes available and the lactic acid can be cleared, allowing continued exercise.

Longer-lasting events are fuelled by aerobic energy systems, which use oxygen. Different energy-providing substances in the body are broken down to release their energy, including glycogen stored in the muscle and liver, glucose from the blood, fatty acids from the blood, and stored fat and amino acids from muscle, blood, liver and the gut. The metabolism of these substances provides most of the energy needed for events lasting from three minutes to three hours and beyond. Because the rate of exercise in these instances is less intense, oxygen becomes available to the working muscle, allowing the body to use more of the aerobic systems and less of the anaerobic systems.

SWITCHING SYSTEMS

When you start exercising, the first few minutes can seem exhausting, especially if you start at a high intensity, but gradually, as you take in more oxygen, there is a switch from the anaerobic to the aerobic systems and you are able to tolerate the exercise, or even increase the intensity. The crossover from anaerobic to aerobic is determined by many factors, including the intensity and duration of the exercise and the fitness level of the athlete, as well as prior nutrient intake and energy stores. An untrained individual who goes for a first run will struggle to make it a mile without stopping, as anaerobic systems dominate, but with training comes a more frequent and efficient use of aerobic systems, allowing the runner to continue comfortably for as long as they desire.

ABOVE: Endurance exercise such as long-distance swimming will be fuelled by a combination of glycogen and fatty acids.

OPPOSITE LEFT: The more you train, the more efficient your body becomes at switching fuel systems.

OPPOSITE RIGHT: Gadgets can monitor your heart rate and the amount of calories burned.

ENERGY FOR EXERCISE

If a person is working out at a high intensity – at around 70% of their maximal oxygen capacity for an hour or longer – approximately 50% of the energy used up will come from carbohydrate. This exertion is the equivalent of a well-trained runner running a marathon or half marathon at a pace of around seven minutes per mile (four minutes per km) – in other words, not talking pace. The remaining energy is derived from the oxidation of fatty acids – those already in the bloodstream and also those mobilized from fat stores. As the intensity of the exercise decreases, for example to a pace where a conversation could be held, less carbohydrate is used up and fat becomes the principal energy source.

Training does not alter the total amount of energy expended for a given event but rather the proportion of energy derived from carbohydrates and fat changes with the intensity of the exercise. As a person becomes fitter aerobically, the body is able to adapt, and the energy derived from fat increases and that derived from carbohydrates decreases. A trained athlete uses a greater percentage of fat than an untrained person does at the same workload.

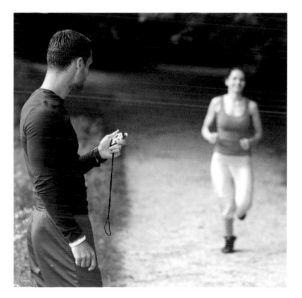

HUNGRY WORK

The difference in fuel usage can help to explain the changes experienced in appetite after exercise. A two-hour walk might use up around 600 calories, but fat would be the dominant fuel source, which has little impact on appetite. An hour's run at a quick pace might also use up 600 calories but carbohydrate would make a significant contribution, and this depletes glycogen stores and can make you feel hungry soon afterwards. For this reason, low-intensity fat-burning exercise is often recommended for weight loss.

EATING FOR VICTORY

The goal of professional and elite athletes is to improve fitness and performance to the maximum of their capabilities, to give them an advantage over their competitors in a world in which a second could be the difference between failure and success, and in which other environmental factors cannot be controlled. For these athletes, meeting energy needs, especially from carbohydrates, becomes a nutrition priority, as optimum athletic performance is promoted by adequate energy intake and the availability of sufficient glycogen.

The goal of most regular exercisers is to become a bit fitter, maybe feel better running up the stairs, and to lose a bit of weight or just maintain the same clothes size. Thus there is a huge difference in how an athlete should eat compared to, say, a fun-runner. However, the principles of sports nutrition and the athletic diet have filtered down into the mainstream media and specially designed products such as gels and drinks are available to all. Mistakenly, people who want to get fit think they should start eating like an athlete.

DOES EVERYBODY NEED TO CARB-LOAD?

If you eat a typical mixed diet, your body has the capacity to store 350–500g (12–18oz) of glycogen, which is more than enough to get you through a session in the gym or a 10k (six-mile) run. This means that grabbing a banana or energy bar pre-workout is often completely unnecessary.

FOR EVENTS LASTING LONGER than 90 minutes, it is thought that taking on extra energy a short time beforehand could be useful in aiding performance; for endurance events such as marathons or four-hour cycle stages, carb-loading has been recommended. This is the practice of allowing your glycogen stores to deplete for a few days in advance of the event by eating a low-carb diet and then eating big quantities of carbohydrate foods in the 48 hours before the event. The idea is that this prevents a person "hitting the wall", which occurs when an athlete depletes their limited reserves of glycogen and the body is forced to use fatty acids and amino acids as sources of energy. These cannot be metabolized as quickly as glycogen so the body is forced to slow down, which causes the athlete to slow down quite dramatically too. Runners seldom hit the wall in races of half-marathon distance and less, but it can be more common in marathons, especially if their pace is fast.

However, scientists are now debating the necessity of this carb-loading, as there are other strategies that may be more useful in avoiding complete glycogen depletion. Furthermore, glycogen depletion varies widely among those taking part in endurance events: some runners hit the wall earlier than others, and some don't hit it at all – and among those runners who don't experience the wall, some are able to maintain much faster paces than others. Therefore it would seem that glycogen depletion is highly individual, which challenges the blanket advice about carb-loading.

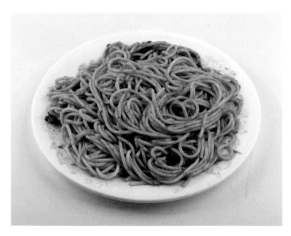

LEFT: A big plate of spaghetti is often the meal of choice the night before an endurance event.

OPPOSITE: A micrograph of glycogen (bright pink), which is carbohydrate stored in the muscles and the liver.

TRUST ME, I'M A DIETICIAN
Carb-load the right way

If you are training for an endurance event, such as a marathon or triathlon, the most important thing you can do is to practise your nutrition strategy. Whether you decide to carb-load or rely on gels and sports bars to get you through is up to you; the critical thing is that you know your strategy will work because you have tried and tested it. If you do want to carb-load you should start to build up your carbohydrate intake 48 hours before a long run, swim or bike ride. Choose refined carbs such as white rice or pasta as you do not want to fill yourself up with too much fibre – this could prevent you eating enough carbohydrate and may have unwanted side effects on your bowel.

Avoid rich creamy sauces and large portions of protein as again these will be filling. A typical daily menu could include a bowl of cereal with toast and jam or mashed banana, a baked potato with tuna and sweetcorn and a large bowl of pasta with a chicken and tomato sauce; snack in between on cereal bars, yogurt, pancakes and scones. Practise this for five to six weeks for your long training runs and you will be able to gauge if you are getting your portion sizes and snacks right depending on how you feel while training. Finally, the night before the actual event stick to the plan, don't stuff yourself and get up early and have your usual breakfast.

STORAGE CAPACITY

The distance a runner can run or a cyclist can cycle before glycogen depletion occurs depends on how much glycogen they can store and how fast the glycogen is being used up. The liver stores approximately 100g (3.5oz) of glycogen, with the rest being stored in muscles. Training greatly increases an athlete's glycogen-storage capacity and carb-loading is able to exploit that capacity.

However, it is thought that strategies to spare glycogen are more effective than those designed to maximize storage. Sparing glycogen can be achieved in two ways. First, endurance athletes can follow specialized training plans to allow adaptations to occur in the muscles. This is known as "training low", whereby the athlete follows a low-carb diet or trains in the fasted state, i.e. on an empty stomach, which encourages the muscle fibres to become more efficient at using fatty acids as a fuel source.

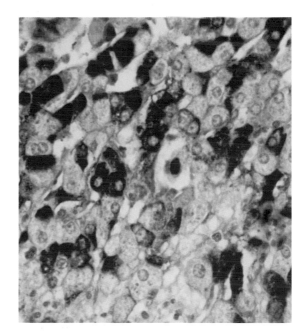

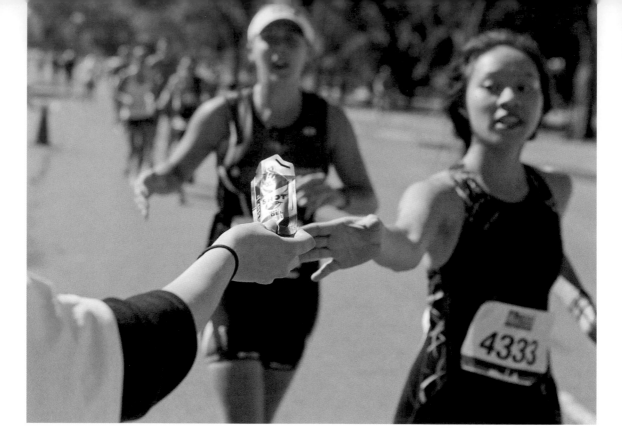

This means that when they are competing, the muscles will be able to use more fatty acids, thus sparing glycogen and making the stores last throughout the event. The second strategy is to consume fast-acting carbohydrates during the event. Studies have shown that this can replace approximately a third of the glycogen being used up at heart rates around 80% of maximum. One study looked at the performance of athletes with either high or low initial glycogen levels, and who either did or did not take on carbohydrate during the trial. They found that the athletes performed just as well when they started with low glycogen levels and consumed carbs during the event as when they started with high glycogen levels and did not consume carbs. The athletes didn't perform any better when they started with high glycogen levels and consumed carbs during the trial.

ABOVE: Replacing energy while you run could negate the need to carb-load the day before.

RIGHT: Energy bars and gels are popular and convenient for runners and cyclists but a handful of sweets could be just as effective.

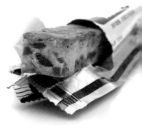

The bottom line: For certain athletes in certain races, carb-loading can make a difference, even with carbohydrate consumption during the event, so the best advice is that they practise their strategy pre-race. For the majority of us, however, carb-loading is wholly unnecessary.

IS HIGH-INTENSITY BETTER THAN ENDURANCE?

It seems that anyone involved in the fitness industry is raving about the benefits of high-intensity interval training (HIIT). This method of training involves repeated bouts of high-intensity exercises that typically last for 40 seconds, followed by a 20-second rest, but which can range from five seconds to eight minutes, followed by recovery periods of varying lengths, depending on the exercise.

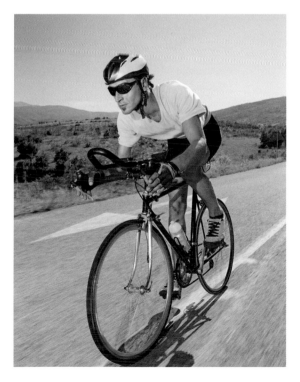

THERE IS GOOD REASON for HIIT to have become so popular, as scientists have demonstrated that it improves both the fitness and performance of professional athletes and recreational exercisers alike, and may achieve the same fitness benefits that result from endurance training or continuous aerobic exercise.

Traditionally it was thought that endurance exercise, such as long-distance running or cycling, was the best way to improve cardiovascular fitness. While these regimes could confer benefits to the heart, they often increase the risk of injury and strain on the working muscles and tendons. Current research has compared different markers of fitness and shown that HIIT can improve them to a similar degree to high-volume continuous exercise – and in less time. So should we all be abandoning cycling and swimming for short bursts of HIIT?

LEFT: Endurance activities such as cycling have long been used to improve cardiovascular fitness.

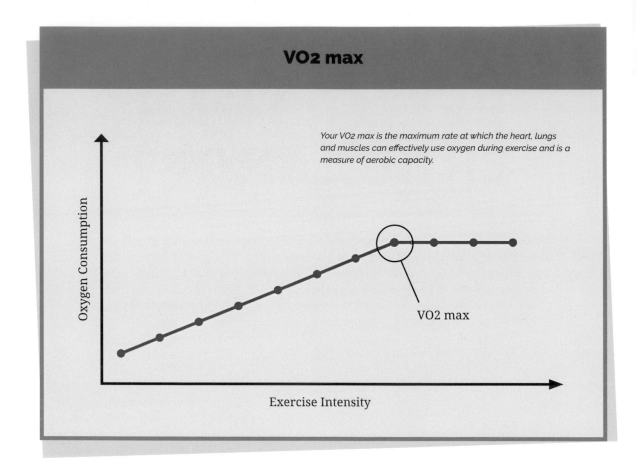

VO2 max

Your VO2 max is the maximum rate at which the heart, lungs and muscles can effectively use oxygen during exercise and is a measure of aerobic capacity.

Oxygen Consumption

VO2 max

Exercise Intensity

MEASURES FOR FITNESS

Two of the main physiological parameters that are used as a measure of fitness are VO2 max and cardiac function. VO2 max is the maximum oxygen (O2) consumption of an individual during exercise: a measure of their physical fitness as well as an important determinant of their endurance capacity. Research suggests that HIIT exercise results in similar or even superior VO2 max compared with endurance exercise.

Numerous studies have shown that heart function improves with endurance training as the heart muscle thickens and increases in size, but recent work shows that the cardio responses to HIIT are similar – and in some cases superior – to those of

continuous endurance training. One study compared two groups of runners and showed that those who did interval training three days per week for eight weeks had a 10% greater improvement in a marker of cardio fitness compared to the group that ran long and slow distances.

BURNING FAT

Many people who regularly exercise are interested in weight management so an important consideration for choosing one type over the other would be which is better for weight loss – and particularly which burns more fat for fuel during exercise.

Because of the nature of high-intensity exercise, it can be assumed that carbohydrate would be the dominant fuel source, which would not necessarily aid fat loss (and in fact could result in stimulating the appetite through depleted glycogen stores). However, it has been shown that the body quickly adapts to using more fat as a fuel source with regular HIIT sessions; one study showed that, after six weeks of interval training, fat-burning was significantly higher and carbohydrate oxidation significantly lower. This compares favourably against results observed with continuous endurance exercise.

An important benefit of endurance training is the increase in post-exercise energy expenditure, known as Excess Post-exercise Oxygen Consumption (EPOC). After exercising, oxygen consumption does not return to normal levels until the muscle cells are fully recovered. This can last for an hour or so after the session has finished. The elevated level of oxygen consumption increases energy expenditure, so the person burns more calories even though they are resting. Again, a review of the research shows that HIIT results in high EPOC values and compares favourably against endurance exercise.

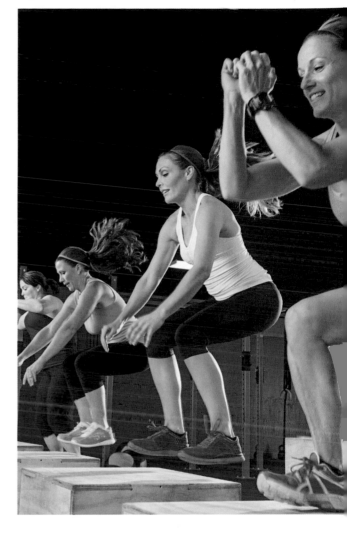

RIGHT: After exercise, oxygen consumption can remain high, burning more calories.

The bottom line: Given the positive outcomes of HIIT in improving not only cardiovascular but also metabolic and skeletal health, it would seem that HIIT can be hailed as a time-efficient, attractive replacement for hours spent pounding the pavement. However, it is important to note that, to be truly effective, HIIT must be performed at the appropriate level of intensity and frequency. It is not easy to "cheat" on endurance exercise – a time or distance goal is set and usually achieved – but during HIIT it is very easy for performance to drop off from 90% maximum heart rate to 70% maximum heart rate as the level of discomfort grows. Rather than pick one type of exercise over the other, incorporating a balance of the two into cardiovascular training allows exercise enthusiasts to reach their goals in the most successful manner.

DOES EXERCISE MAKE YOU LOSE OR GAIN WEIGHT?

When the topic of exercise is raised while counselling weight-loss clients, a common excuse I hear is that they don't exercise because exercise makes them fatter. It's much more likely, given the sort of treats most people like to indulge in after exercise, that they overestimate the number of calories burned during exercise and underestimate the number of calories consumed from the treat. Jogging for 40 minutes may burn around 400 calories, but a "reward" of a takeaway later will result in the consumption of far more calories than if the run had never happened!

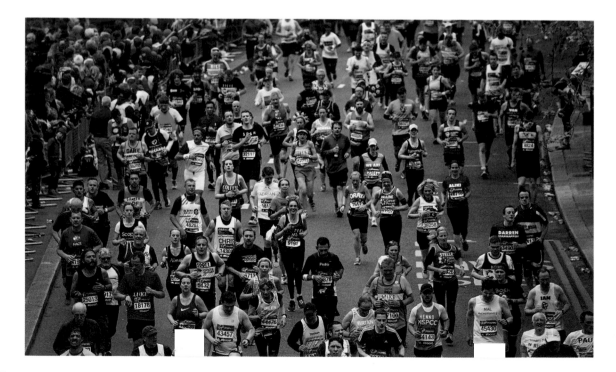

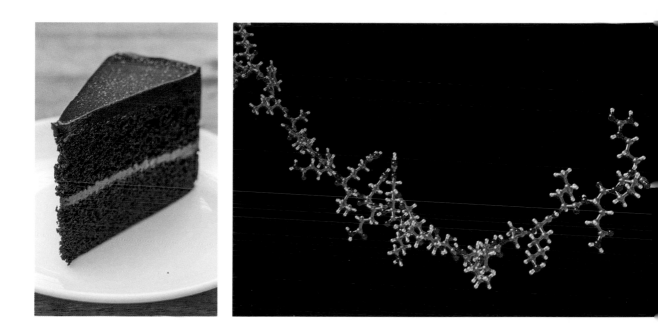

SO WHILE IT CAN'T be claimed that exercise makes you fat, it is a common misconception that exercise (without an accompanying diet) will lead to weight loss. Every year, a local charity asks me to give a nutrition talk to their fundraising runners in the lead-up to the London Marathon, and each time I warn them: don't expect to lose weight. Many would-be marathon runners are under the illusion that they will shed weight during training, but then experience the complete opposite and gain weight. A small part of this gain will be due to an increase in muscle, but mainly it will be through an imbalance of calories in versus calories out. Getting up early for long runs demands an increase in calorie intake, but calorie expenditure can easily be matched and even surpassed through energy drinks, snacks before and after the run, bigger breakfasts and then the treat slice of cake to reward the effort.

But while it is much easier to lose weight through dietary changes alone – and, conversely, exceedingly difficult to achieve the same weight loss just with exercise – that does not equate to exercise making you fat.

EXERCISE AND APPETITE

Exercise can both suppress appetite and stimulate hunger. It's very common to not feel like eating for a good hour or so after a particularly strenuous session, but a few hours later it's likely you'll feel ravenous. Research has shown that, following vigorous exercise, there is an increase in the level of a hormone known as peptide YY. This has the effect of reducing the level of the appetite-stimulating hormone known as ghrelin. As time passes, however, levels of peptide YY will drop, allowing appetite to develop. Research also shows that exercise increases levels of insulin and leptin, both of which are appetite-stimulating hormones.

....

OPPOSITE: The average runner will burn about 100 calories per mile (60 calories per km) during a marathon.

ABOVE LEFT: If you reward yourself with cake every time you exercise, you are unlikely to lose weight.

ABOVE RIGHT: Grehlin is known as the "hunger hormone" and is involved in the regulation of appetite.

TRUST ME, I'M A DIETICIAN
How to exercise

In terms of exercise, it is recommended we do "five a week"; this is translated from the official WHO recommendation that adults aim to exercise for a total of 150 minutes per week. Despite the "five a week" catchphrase, it is not recommended that we do 5 x 30 minutes of the same exercise, but rather that we vary the length and intensity of the exercise and incorporate two sessions of muscle-strengthening activities, such as circuit training. The exercise doesn't have to be done in one go: the message is to become more active generally, rather than to offset a sedentary lifestyle with bursts of exercise.

It is important not to downplay the benefits of exercise. The part it plays in weight loss has been overstated, but it plays a crucial role in most aspects of our physical health, in fighting disease and in moderating mental health.

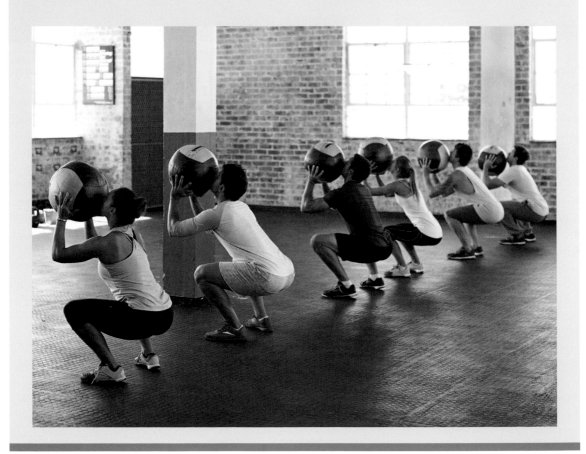

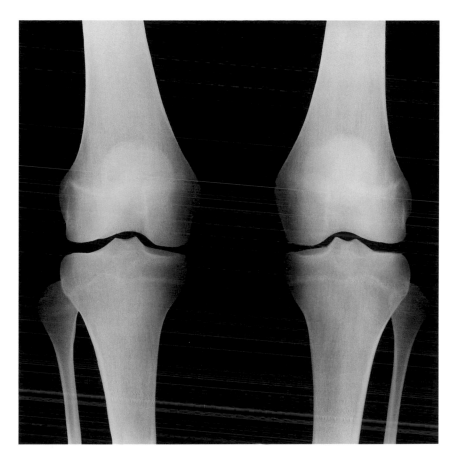

OPPOSITE: The exercise recommendation for adults is five 30-minute sessions per week of a combination of cardio and strength workouts.

LEFT: Look after your knees! Exercise is important in protecting and strengthening the joints.

STAYING ACTIVE

Another reason exercise may not lead to weight loss is the compensation of being less physically active afterwards. So, for instance, the long run you do at 6 a.m. may mean you are more likely to take things easy for the rest of the day. This was the explanation offered by researchers who investigated the effect of exercise on weight loss on a large group of overweight women. The women were divided into four groups. Three of the groups worked out for different lengths of time each week with a personal trainer, and the control group remained inactive. The women were asked to stick to their usual diets. Those who exercised did not lose significantly more weight than the inactive participants. They did reduce their waist measurements a little, but lost no more body fat overall than the control group.

The bottom line: Regular exercise is a critical part of a maintaining good health. The benefits include keeping muscles and joints healthy, improving sleep, reducing risk of depression and anxiety, and promoting self-esteem. Exercise impacts on appetite but does not cause overeating or weight gain. While it can help maintain a healthy weight, it is not a significant solution to the quest for weight loss.

SHOULD YOU ALWAYS TRAIN WITH A SPORTS DRINK?

At my boot-camp sessions I see half the class with a bottle of something orange or purple and the others, like me, with just a bottle of water. The correct choice depends on the intensity and duration of the workout. Water is generally sufficient for shorter sessions (like boot camp), but for exercise lasting more than 60 minutes an isotonic sports drink could be recommended.

It can be argued that sports drinks are useful for shorter workouts. Those who exercise first thing in the morning on an empty stomach, for example, may feel hungry and find a sports drink helps take the edge off. For high-intensity exercise a sports drink will provide readily available energy, but it is likely the body will have sufficient glycogen stores to provide this energy if the individual is eating a normal mixed diet. A sports drink is unlikely to make much difference to the typical recreational runner, whose slower pace means that fat will be the predominant fuel source.

Sports drinks provide two key ingredients, carbohydrate and sodium. The carbohydrate provides fuel for working muscles and the sodium is an electrolyte that helps to maintain fluid balance. Some sports drinks also provide other electrolytes, such as potassium and chloride, small amounts of which are lost in sweat. However, there are

different drink formulations to choose from, including isotonic, hypertonic and hypotonic. An isotonic drink (such as Lucozade Sport or Gatorade) contains 6–8% carbohydrate solution, which has the effect of enabling rapid absorption; this formulation has been shown to be absorbed into the body more rapidly than water. Isotonic solutions use artificial sweeteners to improve palatability, as the solution itself is not pleasant-tasting; studies have shown that athletes won't consume enough of a sports drink of which they don't like the taste.

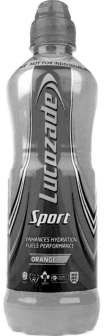

Hypotonic drinks contain a less concentrated carbohydrate solution (1–3%), which promotes water absorption but provides less carbohydrate energy and fewer calories than isotonic drinks, while hypertonic drinks have a carbohydrate concentration greater than 10%. These latter have a slow gastric emptying rate and so decrease fluid absorption, which makes them unsuitable for use during exercise but useful post-exercise to aid recovery.

WHAT IS GOOD HYDRATION?

Adequate hydration is crucial for elite and professional athletes as well as for the average jogger or gym member (albeit to a lesser degree).

Being well hydrated is an important consideration for optimal exercise performance. Because dehydration increases the risk of potentially life-threatening heat injury, such as heat stroke, athletes should strive for euhydration (hydration balance) before, during and after exercise. Dehydration (loss of more than 2% body weight) can compromise aerobic exercise performance, particularly in hot weather, and may impair mental and cognitive performance.

HOW TO MAINTAIN GOOD HYDRATION

The reason we sweat when we exercise is that our bodies need to dissipate the heat created. The amount we sweat varies widely between individuals and is dependent on many factors, from the humidity to our body weight and how acclimatized we are to the temperature. Studies show that sweat rates can range from 300 to 2,400ml (10–80fl oz) per hour for different types of exercise performed in different conditions. While the average amount of sodium lost in sweat is approximately 1g (0.035oz) per litre, this also varies widely between individuals; some people, known as "salty sweaters", lose much more sodium in their sweat than others. Many professional sports teams test their athletes in order to identify those with heavier losses of sodium through sweat, so that they can adjust their intakes accordingly.

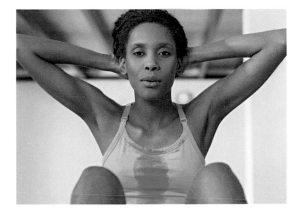

Different sweat rates and poor hydration strategies (too much water, lack of electrolytes) can cause problems such as hyponatraemia or muscle cramps. Hyponatraemia occurs when the blood's sodium concentration sinks too low, which can result from prolonged, heavy sweating without replacing sodium, or from excessive water intake. Hyponatraemia is more likely to develop in novice marathoners who are not lean, who run slowly, who sweat less, or who consume excess water before, during or after the event. Muscle cramps are associated with dehydration, electrolyte deficit and muscle fatigue. They are more common in profuse sweaters who experience large sweat-sodium losses.

BEFORE EXERCISE

To be in the optimum state of hydration (euhydration), it is recommended that an individual drinks around 5–7ml (0.17–0.24fl oz) of fluid per kilogram of body weight about 30–60 minutes before exercise begins. This could be water or an isotonic sports drink.

....

OPPOSITE: Sports drinks have been specially formulated to deliver both hydration and energy.

ABOVE: Sweat loss can lead to dehydration which impacts performance.

OVERLEAF: In some sports there are limited opportunities to take on more fluid.

 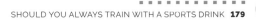

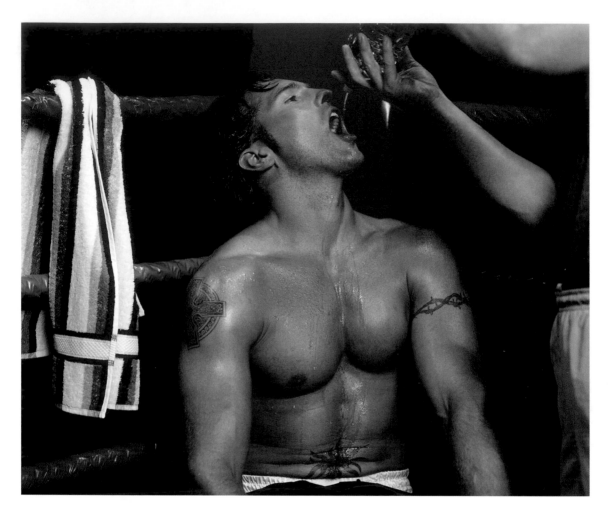

For example, a 70kg (154lb or 11-stone) man should drink 300–500ml (10–17fl oz). This allows him enough time to optimize his hydration status and excrete any excess fluid as urine. Being overhydrated, known as hyperhydration, should be avoided: it not only causes discomfort but also greatly increases the chance of having to pass urine during the event. There is no clear physiological or performance advantage of hyperhydration over euhydration.

DURING EXERCISE

The aim of drinking during exercise is to offset the fluid lost through sweat. However, as sweat loss is highly variable between individuals and will also depend on factors such as temperature, duration and how often there are opportunities to drink, the amount of fluid needed will vary. Runners and cyclists can carry their water, for instance, whereas footballers and boxers must wait for breaks. For this reason, there is not an official recommendation for the amount or type of fluid to consume.

Athletes should be aware that dehydration is possible even in colder weather, since a significant amount of fluid will still be lost from the body through respiration and sweat will still be lost due to more insulated clothing (such as in skiing).

TRUST ME, I'M A DIETICIAN
Calculating your sweat rate

If you want to work out sweat rate, you should use a heavy training session in which you know you will sweat but during which you cannot consume any fluids. First, weigh yourself naked before you begin. (Record your weight in kilograms to make the conversion to fluids easier.) After your training session, towel off any sweat and weigh yourself again. The amount of weight lost can be converted to grams by multiplying by 1,000. This figure is equal to the millilitres of fluid lost and is the quantity you should aim to consume when you train.

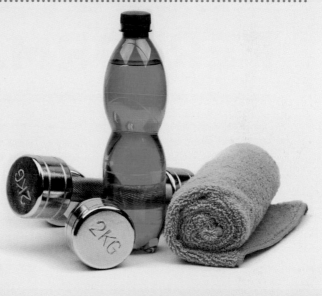

Dehydration can also occur in cold weather because of a reduced incentive to drink, notably not wanting to consume a cold drink, or because of not wanting to remove multiple layers of clothing to urinate.

For events longer than an hour, sports drinks containing 6–8% carbohydrates and some electrolytes can be helpful in replacing fluid and sodium losses and providing energy.

AFTER EXERCISE
Replacing fluids and electrolytes lost through sweat can be achieved by consuming a normal meal and drink after the event has finished. If excessive dehydration has occurred, drinking 500ml of fluid for every half-kilogram (c.1lb) of body weight lost should aid a rapid recovery. Consuming rehydration beverages and salty foods at meals and snacks will help replace fluid and electrolyte losses.

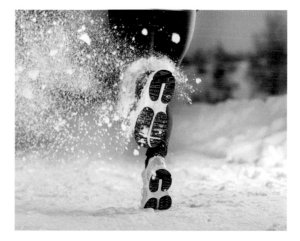

ABOVE: It is possible to become dehydrated even when exercising in cold climates.

WILL SUPPLEMENTS BOOST YOUR PERFORMANCE?

Athletes are always looking for something extra, beyond training and regular diet, to give them the edge. There are a number of substances – some legal, some not so legal – that claim to be able to boost performance. These are known as ergogenic supplements. They work in a variety of ways, from helping to prepare an individual for exercise to improving exercise recovery.

POPULAR ERGOGENIC AIDS INCLUDE caffeine, carnitine and creatine, but controversy surrounds them all. The International Society of Sports Nutrition defines an ergogenic aid as a training or psychological technique, mechanical device, nutritional practice or pharmacological agent that can help improve exercise-performance capacity or enhance physical strength.

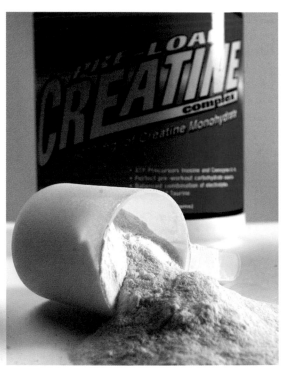

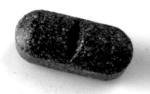

RIGHT: Caffeine (here in pill form) is a popular ergogenic aid that can help endurance.

FAR RIGHT: Creatine can help build muscles and reduce injury.

Ergogenic aid	What is it?	Claim	Evidence	Should I take it?
Caffeine	Naturally occurring substance found in tea and coffee.	Improves endurance performance.	Good. Caffeine is a central-nervous-system stimulant that has been shown to improve focus and reduce perception of effort.	Yes. Try a couple of cups of coffee 30 minutes or so before you exercise, but be aware that too much could cause dizziness and unwanted bowel movements.
Carnitine	Carnitine is a substance made in the body that is needed for energy production.	Because carnitine is needed for the transport of fatty acids to cells where they can be metabolized, it is claimed that, taken as a supplement, it can increase fatty-acid metabolism and aid fat loss.	Weak. Although there is now evidence that it may aid in recovery.	Although there are no reported side effects (from a 2–4g/0.7–1.4oz dose), it is probably not worth it.
Creatine	Creatine is made in the body and has a role in the phospha-gen energy system.	It is popular with bodybuilders and sprinters, who believe it can enhance energy needed for explosive sports.	Fair. Creatine sup-plementation can in-crease muscle mass and allow individuals to train harder. It can also lessen potential for injury.	For the right sport, a dose of 3–5g (0.1–0.17oz) per day could be useful for increasing strength and speed.
Conjugated linoleic acid (CLA)	A type of fatty acid found in the body.	Supplementing CLA increases muscle and bone mass and decreases body fat.	Weak. Some research showed this effect in animal studies but little evidence for the same effect in humans.	No.

Ergogenic aid	What is it?	Claim	Evidence	Should I take it?
Branched-chain amino acids (BCAA)	Branched-chain amino acids are a group of essential amino acids with a similar structure. They include leucine, isoleucine and valine.	Although we get sufficient BCAA from eating a balanced diet, it is thought that taking extra BCAA as a supplement will help to improve strength, power and endurance.	Fair. BCAA have a key role in the repair and strengthening of muscles after exercise. The provision of BCAA at the time of exercise or soon afterwards is thought to be important, as research has shown that levels of BCAA in the blood drop after exercise as they are taken up by the muscles to aid recovery. Decreasing levels of BCAA in the blood have also been linked to fatigue during exercise. Supplementation with BCAA may prevent reduced levels in the blood and potentially prove beneficial during prolonged endurance exercise.	Possibly, though you could just as easily have a glass of milk or another food source of BCAA. However, taking up to four 5g doses per day is considered safe.
Andro/DHEA	Androstenedione (andro) and dehy-droepiandrosterone (DHEA) are prohormones that the body can potentially convert to testosterone.	They are popular with bodybuilders, who believe that boosting testosterone levels will result in increased muscle mass and strength.	None. There is no evidence that prohormones boost muscle mass in young men with normal hormone levels.	Andro: no. Andro is banned under the Anabolic Steroid Control Act. DHEA: no. Although DHEA can be purchased over the counter, its safety and the effect of high doses or long-term use are unknown.

Dietary supplements improve performance

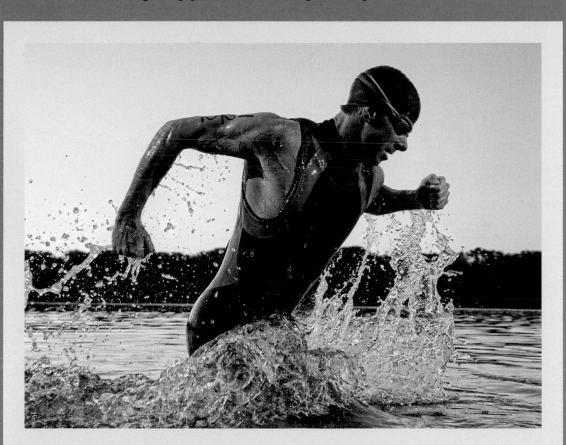

If you get chatting to a serious runner, cyclist or triathlete, the chances are they will be taking a supplement of some type, be it a multivitamin or a herbal remedy. And they will cite myriad reasons for its use, from helping with a niggling injury to boosting energy and performance.

It is true that many vitamins are involved in the biological processes important for exercise and that the more you exercise, the greater demand there is by the body. For example, many of the B vitamins are involved in processing carbohydrate and fat for energy production, and they are also essential to the formation of haemoglobin in red blood cells, which in turn is needed to deliver oxygen to the muscles during aerobic endurance exercise. It is also true that vitamin deficiencies will impair exercise performance. However, what is not true is that you cannot get the extra vitamins you need from your diet alone; in fact, most studies report that if you are meeting your energy needs through a higher-calorie diet, as long as that diet is balanced you will be able to meet your requirements for any extra nutrients you need.

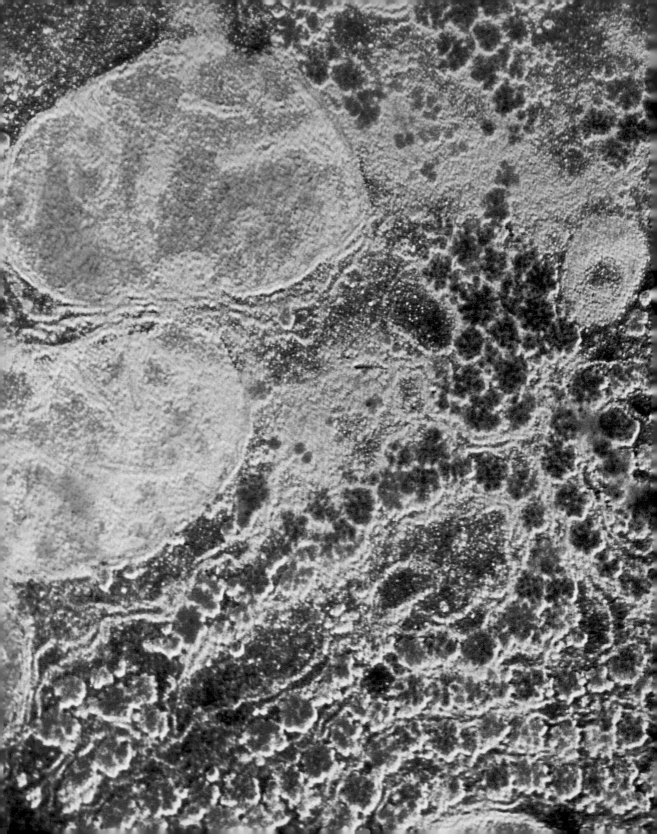

A section through a human liver cell, in which glycogen (shown in pink) is stored.

GLOSSARY

Aerobic exercise Low-to high-intensity exercise in which oxygen is used to generate energy. Also known as cardio.

Amino acids Molecules that join together in chains to form proteins. Often referred to as building blocks.

Anaemia A condition in which blood does not contain enough red blood cells. Iron-deficiency anaemia can be caused by a lack of iron in the diet.

Anaerobic exercise Short-duration, intense exercise powered by metabolic processes that do not use oxygen.

Antibodies Proteins that are used by the body's immune system to identify and neutralize pathogens.

Antigens Chemicals that are foreign to the body and cause an immune response.

Antioxidants Molecules that protect cells from damage caused by the oxidation of other molecules.

Atwater factors A measure of the availability of energy from nutrients, as determined by the Atwater system.

BMR Basal metabolic rate, the minimum amount of energy that is needed to keep the body functioning at rest.

Calcium A mineral needed by the body to maintain strong teeth and bones and to help it to perform such functions as blood clotting and muscle contraction.

Calorie A unit of energy used for food. Specifically, the amount of energy needed to raise the temperature of 1g of water by 1°C. In everyday use, "calorie" usually refers to a kilocalorie (1,000 calories).

Carbohydrate A group of organic compounds comprising sugars, starches and fibres. The body's main source of energy.

Coeliac disease A lifelong condition in which the ingestion of gluten causes damage to the small intestine and inhibits the absorption of nutrients.

Dehydration A state in which the loss of bodily fluids exceeds the amount taken in.

DIAAS Digestible indispensable amino acid score. A measure of protein quality.

Electrolyte Chemicals found in bodily fluids that perform important functions. Examples include calcium, sodium and potassium.

Energy balance The relationship between energy taken into the body and energy being used in the body.

EPOC Excess post-exercise oxygen consumption. The amount of oxygen needed to restore the body to its normal metabolic level.

Ergogenic aids A substance or treatment used to enhance sporting performance.

Euhydration A normal state of hydration.

Fatty acids Molecules found in fats and oils.

Fibre A complex carbohydrate that cannot be digested by the body. Important for increasing the bulk of stools and maintaining healthy digestion.

Free sugars Simple sugars added to foods by manufacturers and naturally present in honey, fruit juices and syrups.

GI Glycaemic index. A rating system that describes the ability of a food to raise blood glucose levels.

Gluten A protein found in wheat and related grains.

Glycogen A storage molecule of glucose. Found in the liver and in muscles.

Ghrelin A hormone that drives appetite, produced in the stomach and pancreas.

HIIT High-intensity interval training, comprised of short periods of intense anaerobic exercise.

Iron An essential mineral necessary for the transport of oxygen in the body.

Isoflavones Plant-based compounds similar in chemical structure and function to oestrogen.

Lactase An enzyme that breaks down lactose.

Lactic acid A chemical that accumulates in the muscles when oxygen levels in the body are low. Responsible for a burning sensation in active muscles.

Lactose A sugar found in milk and dairy products.

LDL-cholesterol Low density lipoprotein cholesterol, or "bad cholesterol", forms the majority of the body's cholesterol.

Metabolism All the chemical reactions in the body necessary to maintain life. Includes growth and repair, cell renewal and movement.

Monounsaturated fat Fatty acids that contain a single double bond and are liquid at room temperature.

Obesogenic An environment in which people are encouraged to eat unhealthily and perform little exercise.

Oestrogen The group of hormones that are reponsible for the female characteristics of the body.

Omega-3 A group of polyunsaturated fatty acids that have their first double bond at the third carbon in the chain and have been shown to confer health benefits.

Osteoporosis A condition that affects the bones, making them brittle and fragile.

Pathogen Any microorganism that causes disease or illness.

Peptide YY A hormone produced in the small intesine that reduces appetite.

Polyunsaturated fat Fatty acids that have more than one double bond and are dominant in plant-based foods and oils.

Probiotics Live bacteria and yeasts belived to confer health benefits.

Processed food Food that has been altered from its natural state in any way.

Protein A group of organic compounds, made up of chains of amino acids.

Saturated fat Fatty acids that do not contain any double bonds, giving them the property of being solid at room temperature. Often dominant in animal products, such as butter, fatty red meats and full-fat dairy products.

Serotonin A neurotransmitter thought to regulate mood, sometimes called a happiness hormone.

TEF Thermic effect of food, the energy used when your body is digesting and assimilating food.

Trans fat A type of unsaturated fat that is solid at room temperature, found in manufactured products like margarine and deep-fried foods.

Veganism A lifestyle in which all animal-derived products are avoided.

Vitamin B12 A B vitamin necessary for the function of nerves, the brain and red blood cells.

Vitamin C A vitamin that helps the growth of tissue and bones.

Vitamin D A vitamin necessary for bone, teeth and muscle health.

VO2 max The maximum oxygen consumption of an individual during exercise.

Whole food Foods based on whole ingredients, with minimal processing, additives or other artificial substances.

INDEX

CREDITS

The publishers would like to thank the following sources for their kind permission to reproduce the pictures in this book.

Cornell University 50 (top)

Cosmed: 33

Getty Images: Baona 58, Mieke Dalle 12 (top), Roger Harris/Science Photo Library 46 (top), Tony Karumba/AFP 47, Jonathan Kirn 17 (right), David Trood 56, Yellowdog 17 (left)

Science Photo Library: 15, Biophoto Associates 19 (bottom), Burger/Phanie 28, Eye of Science 18, Steve Lowry 86-87, Cordelia Molloy 62 (top), Miriam Maslo 13, Alfred Pasieka 38, Jose Antonio Penas 19 (top), Sciepro 8, Stephanie Schuller/Alistair Walsham 29, Shelia Terry 26, Carol & Mike Werner/Visuals Unlimited, Inc. 12 (bottom)

Shutterstock.com: 1989studio 27, Africa Studios 66 (right), 85, Avatar_023 36, Peter Bernik 53 (top), Bigacis 79 (left), Jose Luis Calvo 54, Andras Csontos 68, Daxiao Productions 46 (bottom), Charlie Edwards 74, Kalin Eftimov 20, Feelplus 41, Yulia Furman 82 (top), Arina P Habich 21, Anna Hoychuk 7, Joseph 71, Karnavalfoto 78, Sebastian Kaulitzki 83, Rob Kints 45, Kateryna Kon 10, Lightpoet 42, Lightspring 76, Malivan Lullia 80 (top), Lzf 30, Natalilia K 50, Robyn Mackenzie 14 (centre), Magdanatka 70, Maks Narodenko 39, Naturalbox 24, Oleksandra Naumenko 14 (bottom), New York Public Library 49, NeydtStock 48, Official 23, Pixologicstudio 35, Ralwel 81, Rawpixel 39 (top), Roberaten 63, 66 (centre left), Science Source 53 (top), Elena Shashkina 69, Somersault1824 32, Staras 40, Stockforliving 62, Anastasia Stoma 68 (centre), Johan Swanepoel 82 (centre), Karen Struthers 67, Syda Productions 53 (bottom), Mykola Mazuryk 61, Y Photo Studio 79 (right), Yunava1 44, VictoriaKh 66 (centre right), Valentyn Volkov 80 (bottom), Wavebreakmedia 55, Slawomir Zelasko 66 (left)

Original illustrations by Phil O'Farrell: www.philofarrell.co.uk

Every effort has been made to acknowledge correctly and contact the source and/or copyright holder of each picture and Carlton Books Limited apologises for any unintentional errors or omissions, which will be corrected in future editions of this book.